Contents

1 Chapter 1: Understanding Disease Remission

Disease remission is more than just the absence of symptoms; it's a complex state where the disease activity is significantly reduced or even halted. Understanding the nuances of remission is crucial because it shapes our expectations, influences treatment decisions, and ultimately affects the quality of life for individuals living with chronic conditions. We often associate remission with cancer, but it's a relevant concept across a wide spectrum of diseases, from autoimmune disorders like rheumatoid arthritis to infectious diseases like HIV. Each disease presents its unique challenges and criteria for defining remission. For example, in rheumatoid arthritis, remission is defined by the absence of joint swelling and pain, along with specific blood markers indicating reduced inflammation, while in HIV, remission may mean achieving an undetectable viral load through antiretroviral therapy. This difference highlights the disease-specific nature of remission and the need for tailored approaches in its definition and management.

Historically, the focus in medicine was primarily on alleviating symptoms and prolonging life, and the concept of achieving a state beyond symptom management was often considered idealistic. This perspective was deeply influenced by the limited understanding of disease mechanisms and the lack of effective treatments. Diseases like tuberculosis, polio, and even many forms of cancer were essentially death sentences. However, the advent of antibiotics, vaccines, and more sophisticated therapies gradually shifted the landscape. We started to see cases where diseases could not only be controlled but also, in some instances, pushed into a state of quiescence. The polio vaccine eradicated the disease in many parts of the world, demonstrating the power of prevention. The introduction of combination chemotherapy for childhood leukemia transformed it from a near-certain fatal condition to a highly treatable one, with many children achieving long-term remission. These successes spurred further research and innovation, leading to a growing recognition of the potential for remission as a realistic goal. From the dark ages where physicians thought imbalances caused disease to now, our perception has shifted, and with the advent of modern science, we can finally achieve remission.

However, achieving lasting remission is far from a straightforward process. Several significant challenges impede progress. One of the most formidable is the inherent complexity of diseases themselves. Many chronic conditions are not caused by a single factor but rather by a complex interplay of genetic predispositions, environmental influences, and lifestyle choices. Untangling these intricate relationships is essential for developing targeted therapies that can effectively induce remission. Furthermore, even when effective treatments are available, patient variability can significantly impact outcomes. Factors such as age, overall health, genetic makeup, and adherence to treatment regimens can all influence the likelihood of achieving and maintaining remission. Personalized medicine, which takes into account individual patient characteristics, is increasingly recognized as a crucial approach for optimizing treatment strategies and improving remission rates. The cost of treatments can be an issue that affect patients as well, and sometimes can be inaccessible based on a nation.

Beyond the scientific and medical hurdles, there are also psychological and social factors that can affect a patient's journey toward remission. The uncertainty and anxiety associated with chronic diseases can take a toll on mental health, making it difficult for patients to adhere to treatment plans and maintain a positive outlook. Social support networks, including family, friends, and support groups, can play a vital role in empowering patients and promoting self-management skills. Addressing the emotional and social needs of patients is therefore an integral part of a holistic approach to achieving lasting remission.

Moreover, we must acknowledge the limitations of current therapeutic approaches. While significant advances have been made, many treatments are still imperfect, and relapse remains a common occurrence. For example, in cancer, even after achieving complete remission, there is always a risk that cancer cells may persist in a dormant state, eventually leading to recurrence. Similarly, in autoimmune diseases, medications may effectively suppress inflammation, but they often do not address the underlying immune system dysregulation, increasing the risk of flares.

To overcome these challenges, a multi-pronged approach is needed. Further research is essential to deepen our understanding of disease mechanisms and identify novel therapeutic targets. Clinical trials are critical for evaluating the safety and efficacy of new treatments and for optimizing existing therapies. Innovations in diagnostic tools, such as advanced imaging techniques and molecular profiling, can enable earlier detection of disease and more precise monitoring of treatment response.

In conclusion, understanding disease remission is not merely about defining a term; it's about embracing a paradigm shift in how we approach chronic diseases. It requires a commitment to addressing the complexity of disease, acknowledging patient variability, and recognizing the limitations of current treatments. By fostering collaboration between researchers, clinicians, and patients, and by investing in innovation and personalized medicine, we can pave the way for a future where lasting remission is a reality for more individuals living with chronic conditions. It is a lofty goal, but one that is worth striving for, as it represents the ultimate triumph over disease and a significant step toward improving human health and well-being. Ultimately, remission is not just a scientific concept; it's a beacon of hope for individuals and families affected by chronic diseases, promising a future where they can live full and meaningful lives, free from the burden of illness. And that's what we should aim for: bringing back health for millions.

1.1 Defining Remission in Modern Medicine

Remission, a term resonating with hope and perseverance, represents a pivotal concept in the landscape of modern medicine. It's not simply the absence of disease, but rather a state where the symptoms and signs of a condition are either significantly reduced or have completely disappeared. This concept, however, is far from static; its definition and interpretation have evolved substantially alongside our growing understanding of disease mechanisms and therapeutic interventions. What constitutes remission depends heavily on the specific disease in question, its natural history, and the available tools for diagnosis and monitoring.

In the context of cancer, for instance, remission might signify the absence of detectable tumor cells following treatment. This can be further categorized into complete remission, where there is no evidence of disease, and partial remission, where there is a significant reduction in tumor size or disease burden. Crucially, remission in cancer does not necessarily equate to cure. Microscopic disease may still be present, which can potentially lead to relapse in the future. The duration of remission is therefore a critical factor, with longer periods of remission often associated with a greater likelihood of long-term control. This nuanced understanding necessitates continuous monitoring and follow-up care, even when a patient is considered to be in remission.

Beyond oncology, the concept of remission finds application in a wide array of chronic diseases. In autoimmune disorders like rheumatoid arthritis or multiple sclerosis, remission implies a state of minimal disease activity. Patients in remission might experience few or no symptoms, such as joint pain or neurological deficits, and laboratory markers of inflammation may be within normal ranges. Achieving remission in these conditions often involves the use of immunosuppressive medications to dampen the immune system's attack on the body's own tissues. However, as with cancer, remission in autoimmune diseases can be fragile, and flares of disease activity can occur even after prolonged periods of quiescence. This highlights the importance of ongoing management and lifestyle modifications to maintain remission and prevent relapse.

Moreover, in mental health, remission is a goal in managing conditions like depression or bipolar disorder. It signifies a period where the individual experiences a significant reduction in symptoms, allowing them to function normally and engage in daily activities. Remission in mental health is not simply feeling "better"; it represents a sustained period of stability and well-being. Achieving and maintaining remission often requires a combination of medication, psychotherapy, and lifestyle changes, such as regular exercise and a healthy diet. Relapse is a common concern in mental health, and therefore, ongoing support and monitoring are essential to prevent recurrence of symptoms.

The complexities of defining remission extend further when considering the subjective nature of some disease symptoms. Pain, fatigue, and cognitive dysfunction, for example, are often difficult to quantify objectively. In such cases, remission may be defined based on the patient's self-reported experience and their ability to function in daily life. This emphasizes the importance of patient-centered care and shared decision-making in determining the goals of treatment and assessing the success of interventions. Furthermore, the increasing use of patient-reported outcome measures (PROMs) in clinical trials and routine care is helping to standardize the assessment of subjective symptoms and to better define remission in a patient-relevant manner.

I believe it's essential to acknowledge that the definition of remission can also be influenced by advancements in diagnostic technology. As we develop more sensitive and precise methods for detecting disease, our understanding of what constitutes remission evolves. For example, the advent of minimal residual disease (MRD) testing in leukemia has allowed us to detect very low levels of cancer cells that were previously undetectable. This has led to a redefinition of complete remission in some types of leukemia, with MRD negativity now being considered a more stringent criterion for remission. Similarly, advances in imaging techniques, such as PET scans and MRI, have improved our ability to detect early signs of disease recurrence, allowing for earlier intervention and potentially preventing relapse.

Another aspect to consider is the heterogeneity of disease. Even within a single disease category, such as breast cancer or rheumatoid arthritis, there can be significant variability in the underlying biology and clinical presentation. This heterogeneity makes it challenging to define remission in a uniform way across all patients. Precision medicine approaches, which aim to tailor treatment to the individual characteristics of each patient, are becoming increasingly important in addressing this challenge. By identifying specific biomarkers or genetic profiles that predict response to treatment, we can better define remission in a personalized manner and optimize therapeutic strategies for each patient.

Finally, it's important to recognize that the concept of remission is not without its limitations. While achieving remission is undoubtedly a positive outcome, it's crucial to avoid creating unrealistic expectations. Remission is not a guarantee of cure, and it does not necessarily eliminate the risk of future complications. Patients in remission may still experience long-term side effects from treatment or may require ongoing monitoring and management. Furthermore, the focus on achieving remission should not overshadow the importance of improving quality of life, even in the absence of complete remission. Palliative care and supportive therapies can play a vital role in alleviating symptoms, improving functional status, and enhancing the overall well-being of patients with chronic diseases, regardless of their remission status. The journey towards remission, therefore, requires a holistic approach that addresses the physical, emotional, and social needs of the individual.

Modern medicine defines remission as a multifaceted goal, shaped by disease-specific criteria, technological advancements, and patient-centered considerations. Its ongoing evolution ensures that it remains a relevant and meaningful concept in the pursuit of better health outcomes.

1.2 Historical Perspectives on Disease Trends

Throughout history, the perception and understanding of disease have undergone profound transformations, directly influencing treatment strategies and the very concept of remission. Examining these historical trends offers valuable context for our current pursuits in achieving lasting disease remission. Early civilizations often attributed illnesses to supernatural causes, such as divine punishment or malevolent spirits. Treatment, therefore, revolved around appeasing the gods through rituals, sacrifices, and herbal remedies believed to possess magical properties. The ancient Egyptians, for example, documented their medical practices on papyri like the Ebers Papyrus, which detailed various ailments and their corresponding treatments. While these approaches lacked a scientific basis, they represented early attempts to understand and manage disease within the framework of their beliefs. Remission, in this context, was often viewed as a sign of divine favor or the successful exorcism of evil forces.

The emergence of the classical Greek era marked a significant shift towards a more rational approach to medicine. Hippocrates, considered the "father of medicine," emphasized observation, diagnosis, and prognosis. The Hippocratic Corpus, a collection of medical texts attributed to Hippocrates and his followers, advocated for naturalistic explanations of disease, rejecting supernatural causes. His emphasis on physis, or the body's natural healing power, highlighted the importance of lifestyle and environment in maintaining health. Although Hippocrates didn't explicitly use the term "remission," his writings implied the possibility of recovery and the return to a state of equilibrium in the body. This period saw the development of rudimentary diagnostic tools and therapeutic interventions, such as bloodletting and dietary modifications, based on the humoral theory that posited an imbalance of bodily fluids as the cause of disease. The focus, albeit limited by the scientific understanding of the time, started to shift towards actively influencing the disease process.

The Roman Empire, building upon Greek foundations, further advanced medical knowledge through public health initiatives and the establishment of hospitals. Galen, a prominent Roman physician, synthesized Greek medical knowledge and incorporated his own anatomical and physiological observations. His writings dominated Western medicine for centuries, emphasizing the importance of anatomy and the role of the physician in restoring the body's natural balance. However, the fall of the Roman Empire led to a period of decline in scientific inquiry and a resurgence of supernatural explanations for disease during the Middle Ages. Monasteries became centers of medical knowledge, preserving and translating ancient texts. Medical practices largely consisted of herbal remedies, prayer, and reliance on saints for healing. The concept of remission, while still present, was often intertwined with religious beliefs and viewed as an act of divine intervention rather than a result of medical intervention.

The Renaissance and the Scientific Revolution brought about a renewed emphasis on observation, experimentation, and anatomical study. The invention of the printing press facilitated the dissemination of medical knowledge, and the development of the microscope revolutionized the understanding of the microscopic world. Physicians like Andreas Vesalius challenged Galenic anatomy through detailed dissections, paving the way for a more accurate understanding of human physiology. William Harvey's discovery of blood circulation further revolutionized medical thought, demonstrating the dynamic and interconnected nature of the body. The germ theory of disease, proposed by Louis Pasteur and Robert Koch in the 19th century, revolutionized our understanding of infectious diseases. This breakthrough led to the development of vaccines and antibiotics, which dramatically reduced the incidence and severity of infectious diseases and significantly improved the prospects of achieving remission or complete cure.

The 20th and 21st centuries have witnessed unprecedented advances in medical technology and scientific understanding. The development of sophisticated diagnostic tools, such as X-rays, CT scans, and MRI, has enabled physicians to visualize the body in greater detail and diagnose diseases earlier and more accurately. The advent of molecular biology and genetics has provided insights into the underlying mechanisms of disease at the molecular level. This has led to the development of targeted therapies, such as chemotherapy and immunotherapy, which are designed to specifically attack diseased cells while sparing healthy ones. Furthermore, the concept of personalized medicine has emerged, tailoring treatment strategies to the individual patient based on their genetic makeup and other factors. The concept of remission itself has become more nuanced, with distinctions made between partial and complete remission, as well as the duration of remission. The focus has shifted from simply alleviating symptoms to achieving long-term control of the disease and improving the patient's quality of life. The rise of chronic diseases, such as cancer, diabetes, and autoimmune disorders, has presented new challenges in achieving lasting remission. Research efforts are now focused on developing novel therapeutic approaches, such as gene therapy and regenerative medicine, that hold the promise of not only achieving remission but also restoring the body's natural functions. As we look to the future, understanding the historical context of disease trends is crucial for guiding our efforts in developing innovative strategies to achieve lasting disease remission and improve the health and well-being of individuals worldwide.

1.3 Challenges in Achieving Lasting Remission

Sustaining remission presents a formidable challenge, not merely a celebratory conclusion. The initial triumph of achieving remission often obscures the complex landscape that lies ahead, filled with potential pitfalls and subtle shifts in the disease's behavior. This chapter delves into those challenges, moving beyond the initial victory to explore the critical factors that determine whether remission becomes a lasting reality or a temporary reprieve.

One of the most significant hurdles is the inherent heterogeneity of disease. What appears as a unified condition under a microscope can, at the molecular level, be a constellation of subtly different disease subtypes. This diversity means that a therapy effective against one subset might be utterly useless against another, leading to relapse in patients whose disease composition wasn't fully appreciated initially. Furthermore, this heterogeneity isn't static; it evolves over time. Treatment itself can act as a selective pressure, favoring the survival and proliferation of resistant cells, making the disease more aggressive and difficult to treat upon recurrence. Achieving lasting remission requires a proactive strategy of continuously monitoring the disease's molecular profile, anticipating potential shifts, and adapting treatment regimens accordingly.

Minimal residual disease (MRD) represents another significant obstacle. Even when clinical symptoms have disappeared and standard tests show no evidence of disease, a small number of diseased cells can persist, lurking in protected niches within the body. These cells may be undetectable by conventional methods but possess the potential to re-emerge and trigger a full-blown relapse. Detecting and eradicating MRD is therefore crucial for achieving durable remission. Highly sensitive techniques like next-generation sequencing and flow cytometry are increasingly being used to identify these elusive cells, and therapies are being developed to specifically target them, but challenges remain in reliably identifying and eliminating MRD across different disease types and in ensuring that these treatments don't cause unacceptable side effects.

Furthermore, the long-term effects of treatment can themselves pose challenges to maintaining remission. Chemotherapy, radiation, and even targeted therapies can cause lasting damage to healthy tissues and organs, leading to chronic complications that can compromise overall health and quality of life. These late effects can include cardiovascular problems, neurological deficits, secondary cancers, and endocrine dysfunction. Managing these complications requires a multidisciplinary approach involving specialists in cardiology, neurology, endocrinology, and other fields. It also requires a focus on preventative measures, such as lifestyle modifications and regular screening for secondary malignancies. The goal is not only to keep the disease at bay but also to support the patient's overall well-being and prevent the development of new health problems.

Patient adherence to long-term maintenance therapies presents an additional hurdle. Many diseases require ongoing treatment, even after remission has been achieved, to prevent relapse. However, adhering to these regimens can be challenging, especially for patients who are feeling well and may not fully understand the importance of continued therapy. Factors such as side effects, cost, complexity of the regimen, and lack of social support can all contribute to non-adherence. Improving adherence requires a multifaceted approach that includes patient education, simplification of treatment regimens, management of side effects, and the provision of social and emotional support. Open communication between patients and their healthcare providers is essential to address any concerns and ensure that patients are fully engaged in their care.

The immune system's role in maintaining remission is also paramount, yet often overlooked. Many diseases, particularly cancers, can evade immune surveillance and develop mechanisms to suppress the immune response. A robust immune system is critical for recognizing and eliminating any residual disease cells that may persist after initial treatment. Strategies to enhance immune function, such as vaccines, immune checkpoint inhibitors, and adoptive cell therapies, are being explored to bolster the body's natural defenses against relapse. Additionally, lifestyle factors such as diet, exercise, and stress management can significantly impact immune function and contribute to the maintenance of remission. It is critical to consider the individual's immune landscape when designing long-term maintenance plans.

Access to care disparities significantly complicate the landscape of achieving lasting remission. Socioeconomic status, geographic location, and cultural factors can all impact a patient's ability to access the diagnostic tools, treatments, and supportive care needed to maintain remission. Patients from underserved communities may face barriers to timely diagnosis, treatment, and follow-up, leading to poorer outcomes and a higher risk of relapse. Addressing these disparities requires a concerted effort to improve access to care for all patients, regardless of their background or circumstances. This includes increasing funding for research into diseases that disproportionately affect underserved populations, developing culturally sensitive interventions, and expanding access to affordable healthcare services.

Finally, emotional and psychological factors profoundly influence the ability to sustain remission. The experience of having a serious illness can be incredibly traumatic, and many patients struggle with anxiety, depression, and fear of recurrence, even after achieving remission. These emotional and psychological challenges can significantly impact a patient's quality of life and their ability to adhere to treatment regimens. Providing comprehensive psychological support, including counseling, support groups, and stress management techniques, is essential to help patients cope with the emotional challenges of survivorship and improve their overall well-being. A holistic approach to care that addresses not only the physical but also the emotional and psychological needs of patients is crucial for achieving lasting remission.

2 Chapter 2: Cellular Mechanisms of Remission

Cellular processes stand as the unsung heroes in the quest for disease remission, operating at a microscopic level to orchestrate the return to a state of normalcy. Among these mechanisms, apoptosis, or programmed cell death, emerges as a primary player, serving as the body's way of eliminating compromised cells without triggering widespread inflammation. Imagine it as a highly regulated demolition crew, carefully dismantling cells that are either irreparably damaged or have become rogue elements contributing to disease. This process isn't random; it's governed by intricate molecular pathways that act as checkpoints, ensuring that only the intended targets are eliminated. These pathways involve a cascade of enzymes called caspases, which, once activated, initiate a series of events that ultimately lead to the orderly dismantling of the cell. In cancerous conditions, for instance, tumor cells often evade apoptosis, allowing them to proliferate uncontrollably. Therapies designed to reinstate the apoptotic pathways in these cells can be remarkably effective in inducing remission, effectively shrinking tumors and reducing the burden of disease. The success of such therapies hinges on a deep understanding of the specific apoptotic pathways disrupted in each type of cancer, allowing for targeted interventions that selectively eliminate cancer cells while sparing healthy tissues.

Cellular senescence, on the other hand, presents a more complex picture, acting as both a potential driver and inhibitor of disease progression. It's a state where cells cease dividing but remain metabolically active, secreting a cocktail of molecules known as the senescence-associated secretory phenotype (SASP). The SASP can have both beneficial and detrimental effects depending on the context. In some cases, senescent cells can contribute to tissue repair and prevent the proliferation of pre-cancerous cells, acting as a safeguard against uncontrolled growth. However, in other situations, the SASP can promote inflammation, damage surrounding tissues, and even contribute to the development of age-related diseases. The duality of cellular senescence underscores the need for a nuanced approach to targeting these cells therapeutically. While eliminating senescent cells, known as senolysis, has shown promise in certain conditions, such as age-related macular degeneration, it's crucial to consider the potential consequences of disrupting their beneficial roles in other contexts. The development of senomodulators, which aim to modify the SASP rather than eliminate senescent cells altogether, represents a promising avenue for harnessing the therapeutic potential of senescence while minimizing the risk of adverse effects.

Understanding the interplay between apoptosis and cellular senescence is crucial for developing effective strategies to achieve and maintain disease remission. For example, some cancer therapies work by inducing apoptosis in tumor cells, but surviving cancer cells may enter a state of senescence, potentially contributing to relapse later on. Combining pro-apoptotic therapies with senolytics or senomodulators could, therefore, enhance the durability of remission by eliminating both actively dividing and senescent cancer cells. Moreover, targeting the signaling pathways that regulate both apoptosis and senescence could offer a more comprehensive approach to controlling disease progression. Factors such as the tumor suppressor protein p53, for instance, play a critical role in both apoptosis and senescence, making it a potential target for therapeutic intervention. Strategies to restore p53 function in cancer cells could promote apoptosis, prevent uncontrolled proliferation, and modulate the SASP, thereby improving the chances of achieving lasting remission.

Delving deeper into the molecular intricacies of these processes unveils the significance of intracellular signaling pathways, and epigenetic modifications. Intracellular signaling pathways like the PI3K/Akt/mTOR pathway and the MAPK pathway play crucial roles in regulating cell growth, survival, and apoptosis. Dysregulation of these pathways is frequently observed in various diseases, including cancer, contributing to uncontrolled cell proliferation and resistance to therapy. Targeting these pathways with small molecule inhibitors or other therapeutic agents can effectively restore normal cellular function and induce remission. Furthermore, epigenetic modifications, such as DNA methylation and histone acetylation, can alter gene expression patterns without changing the underlying DNA sequence. These modifications can influence the expression of genes involved in apoptosis, senescence, and other cellular processes critical for disease remission. Epigenetic therapies, such as histone deacetylase inhibitors (HDACi) and DNA methyltransferase inhibitors (DNMTi), have shown promise in reversing aberrant epigenetic modifications and restoring normal gene expression in diseased cells. The combination of epigenetic therapies with other treatment modalities, such as chemotherapy or immunotherapy, can enhance their effectiveness and improve the chances of achieving lasting remission.

Considering the extracellular environment of cells adds another layer of complexity to the understanding of cellular mechanisms of remission. The tumor microenvironment, for instance, plays a critical role in cancer progression and resistance to therapy. Factors such as hypoxia, nutrient deprivation, and immune suppression within the tumor microenvironment can promote tumor cell survival and prevent apoptosis. Targeting the tumor microenvironment with therapies that improve oxygenation, enhance nutrient availability, or stimulate immune cell infiltration can improve the effectiveness of other treatments and promote remission. Similarly, in autoimmune diseases, the inflammatory microenvironment can contribute to chronic inflammation and tissue damage. Therapies that target inflammatory cytokines or immune cells within the affected tissues can reduce inflammation and promote remission.

Therefore, cellular mechanisms of remission are multifaceted and involve a complex interplay of intracellular and extracellular factors. Targeting these mechanisms with precision and specificity holds immense promise for achieving lasting remission in a wide range of diseases. Further research is needed to fully elucidate the intricacies of these processes and develop novel therapeutic strategies that can effectively harness their potential. Understanding cellular senescence and apoptosis requires considering the impact of the immune system. Immune cells play a critical role in eliminating senescent cells and promoting apoptosis of diseased cells. Immunotherapies, such as checkpoint inhibitors and CAR T-cell therapy, can enhance the ability of the immune system to target and eliminate diseased cells, leading to remission. The interaction between the immune system and cellular senescence is particularly complex. Senescent cells can secrete factors that attract immune cells, but they can also express immune checkpoint molecules that inhibit immune cell activity. Understanding these interactions is critical for developing immunotherapies that can effectively target senescent cells and promote disease remission.

Ultimately, the journey toward unraveling the cellular mechanisms of remission requires a convergence of diverse scientific disciplines, fostering collaboration among biologists, chemists, clinicians, and engineers. Through meticulous research, technological advancements, and a shared commitment to improving patient outcomes, the promise of durable remission for a multitude of diseases moves closer to realization.

2.1 Apoptosis and Remission Pathways

Apoptosis, often dubbed programmed cell death, stands as a critical cellular process intricately linked to achieving and maintaining disease remission. Unlike necrosis, a chaotic form of cell death triggered by injury or infection, apoptosis follows a highly regulated molecular pathway, ensuring the orderly dismantling of cells without inciting inflammation or damage to surrounding tissues. This distinction is paramount in disease remission, where eliminating diseased cells without provoking an immune overreaction is vital. I learned this after years researching how specific diseases work and how the body acts to make remission.

At the heart of apoptosis lies a cascade of events orchestrated by a family of enzymes known as caspases. These proteases, present in all cells in an inactive form, are activated by various intracellular or extracellular signals, setting off a chain reaction that leads to the controlled disassembly of cellular components. These signals can be triggered by internal cues, such as DNA damage or mitochondrial dysfunction, or by external factors like growth factor withdrawal or the binding of death ligands to cell surface receptors. The intrinsic pathway, initiated by internal stressors, converges on mitochondria, triggering the release of cytochrome c, which in turn activates caspase-9. The extrinsic pathway, on the other hand, is triggered by the binding of death ligands, such as Fas ligand or TNF-alpha, to their respective receptors on the cell surface, directly activating caspase-8. Regardless of the initiation pathway, the activated initiator caspases then activate executioner caspases, such as caspase-3 and caspase-7, which are responsible for dismantling the cell.

Remission, particularly in cancers and autoimmune disorders, often hinges on the successful induction of apoptosis in diseased cells. In cancer, uncontrolled cell proliferation and resistance to apoptosis are hallmarks of the disease. Cancer cells often acquire mutations that disable critical components of the apoptotic machinery, allowing them to evade cell death signals and proliferate unchecked. Restoring the apoptotic potential of cancer cells is therefore a key therapeutic strategy. Chemotherapeutic agents, radiation therapy, and targeted therapies often work, at least in part, by inducing apoptosis in cancer cells. For instance, chemotherapy drugs like cisplatin damage DNA, triggering the intrinsic apoptotic pathway. Targeted therapies, such as inhibitors of the BCL-2 family of proteins (which inhibit apoptosis), can restore the apoptotic sensitivity of cancer cells. I think this is a valuable thing to know for beginners since the whole process is very complex.

Autoimmune disorders, characterized by the immune system attacking the body's own tissues, also involve defects in apoptosis. In healthy individuals, apoptosis plays a crucial role in eliminating autoreactive immune cells, preventing them from attacking self-antigens. However, in autoimmune diseases, this process is often impaired, leading to the survival and proliferation of autoreactive cells. This can occur due to defects in the expression of death ligands or receptors, or due to abnormalities in intracellular signaling pathways that regulate apoptosis. Promoting apoptosis of autoreactive immune cells is therefore a promising therapeutic approach for autoimmune diseases. For example, drugs that target the TNF pathway, which is involved in both inflammation and apoptosis, can be effective in treating autoimmune conditions like rheumatoid arthritis.

But the story doesn't end there. The effective clearance of apoptotic cells is also crucial for preventing inflammation and promoting tissue homeostasis. Dying cells release signals that attract phagocytes, such as macrophages, which engulf and remove the cellular debris. This process, known as efferocytosis, is essential for preventing the release of intracellular contents that can trigger an inflammatory response. Defects in efferocytosis have been implicated in the pathogenesis of various diseases, including atherosclerosis and autoimmune disorders. Therapeutic strategies that enhance efferocytosis may therefore be beneficial in promoting remission and preventing relapse. Moreover, the efficient removal of apoptotic cells can also prevent secondary necrosis, where the dying cells rupture and release their contents, further exacerbating inflammation. This is one of the key points.

Moreover, the role of apoptosis in remission extends beyond the direct elimination of diseased cells. Apoptosis can also modulate the immune response, shaping the balance between tolerance and immunity. Apoptotic cells can release factors that suppress immune cell activation, promoting tolerance to self-antigens. Conversely, under certain conditions, apoptotic cells can also stimulate immune responses, contributing to the clearance of pathogens or tumor cells. The context-dependent effects of apoptosis on the immune system highlight the complexity of this process and the need for a nuanced understanding of its role in different diseases. Scientists have understood over time that it is fundamental to comprehend it.

Cellular senescence, a state of irreversible cell cycle arrest, is another critical cellular mechanism implicated in disease remission. Senescent cells, while no longer dividing, remain metabolically active and secrete a variety of factors, including cytokines, growth factors, and proteases, collectively known as the senescence-associated secretory phenotype (SASP). The SASP can have both beneficial and detrimental effects on the surrounding tissue environment, depending on the specific context. In some cases, the SASP can promote tissue repair and regeneration, while in other cases it can contribute to inflammation, fibrosis, and tumor progression. The balance between these opposing effects determines the overall impact of senescence on disease remission.

In cancer, cellular senescence can act as a tumor suppressor mechanism, preventing the proliferation of damaged or precancerous cells. Cancer cells that undergo senescence may be effectively eliminated from the tumor microenvironment, contributing to tumor regression and remission.

However, the SASP secreted by senescent cancer cells can also promote tumor growth and metastasis by stimulating angiogenesis, recruiting immune cells, and inducing epithelial-mesenchymal transition (EMT). The context-dependent effects of senescence on cancer highlight the need for careful consideration when targeting senescent cells as a therapeutic strategy. I have been following this aspect for years.

In autoimmune diseases, cellular senescence can contribute to chronic inflammation and tissue damage. Senescent immune cells can secrete inflammatory cytokines that exacerbate autoimmune responses, leading to tissue destruction and disease progression. Targeting senescent immune cells may therefore be a promising therapeutic approach for autoimmune diseases. Conversely, senescence can also play a role in resolving inflammation and promoting tissue repair in certain autoimmune contexts. For example, senescent fibroblasts can secrete factors that stimulate collagen production, contributing to wound healing and tissue remodeling. The complex interplay between senescence, inflammation, and tissue repair in autoimmune diseases requires a deeper understanding to develop effective therapeutic strategies.

Developing therapeutic strategies that harness the power of apoptosis and modulate cellular senescence requires a comprehensive understanding of the underlying molecular mechanisms and the context-dependent effects of these processes. Targeting specific components of the apoptotic pathway or modulating the SASP secreted by senescent cells may offer new avenues for achieving and maintaining disease remission. However, it is crucial to consider the potential off-target effects of these therapies and to develop strategies that selectively target diseased cells while sparing healthy tissues. As our understanding of apoptosis and senescence continues to evolve, new and more effective therapeutic approaches are likely to emerge, paving the way for improved outcomes for patients with a wide range of diseases.

2.2 Cellular Senescence: A Key Factor

Cellular senescence, often described as a state of irreversible cell cycle arrest, represents a pivotal, yet complex, element in the intricate puzzle of achieving durable disease remission. It's a cellular process where cells, after a certain number of divisions or exposure to stressors, cease to proliferate but remain metabolically active. Their influence can be paradoxical. On one hand, senescent cells can contribute to the clearing of damaged or precancerous cells, acting as a tumor-suppressive mechanism and paving the way for remission, particularly in the context of cancer. However, on the other hand, their accumulation over time has been implicated in age-related diseases, chronic inflammation, and, ironically, promoting tumor progression and relapse in some instances. Understanding this duality is key to harnessing its potential in our quest for lasting remission.

The role of cellular senescence in disease remission is multifaceted, depending heavily on the specific disease context. In cancer, for example, therapy-induced senescence (TIS) is a common outcome of chemotherapy or radiation. The induction of senescence in cancer cells can effectively halt their uncontrolled proliferation, leading to tumor shrinkage and clinical remission. This is especially evident in certain types of lymphomas and leukemias, where the cytotoxic effects of treatment induce widespread senescence in malignant cells. The immune system, then, can clear the senescent cells. However, it's not always so straightforward. Senescent cells secrete a complex cocktail of factors known as the senescence-associated secretory phenotype (SASP). This SASP includes pro-inflammatory cytokines, growth factors, and matrix metalloproteinases (MMPs) that can have far-reaching effects on the surrounding tissue microenvironment. Depending on the cellular context and the specific components of the SASP, these factors can either promote the elimination of senescent cells by the immune system or, conversely, drive inflammation, angiogenesis (formation of new blood vessels), and even promote the proliferation and metastasis of remaining cancer cells. This delicate balance dictates whether senescence contributes to durable remission or fuels relapse.

Beyond cancer, cellular senescence is also implicated in the remission of other chronic diseases. In fibrotic diseases, such as liver cirrhosis or pulmonary fibrosis, senescent fibroblasts contribute to the excessive deposition of extracellular matrix, leading to organ damage. Inducing senescence in these cells, or specifically targeting and eliminating them (a strategy known as senolysis), has shown promise in preclinical studies for halting disease progression and even promoting tissue regeneration. Similarly, in autoimmune diseases, such as rheumatoid arthritis, senescent immune cells can contribute to chronic inflammation and joint damage. Targeting these senescent immune cells may help to dampen the autoimmune response and induce remission. However, the specific mechanisms by which senescence contributes to these diseases and how best to target it remain areas of active research. I believe more studies are needed in this area.

Given the complex and context-dependent role of cellular senescence, strategies for manipulating it to promote disease remission require careful consideration. The most obvious approach is to induce senescence in diseased cells. This can be achieved through conventional therapies like chemotherapy and radiation, or through targeted therapies that specifically disrupt cell cycle progression. However, as we have seen, inducing senescence is only half the battle. The SASP released by senescent cells can have detrimental effects, so it's crucial to find ways to mitigate these effects. One approach is to combine senescence-inducing therapies with senolytic drugs, which selectively eliminate senescent cells. This strategy has shown promise in preclinical studies for enhancing the efficacy of cancer therapy and preventing relapse. Senolytics are a novel class of drugs that selectively target and kill senescent cells, offering a potential therapeutic approach to selectively remove these cells and mitigate the harmful effects of the SASP. Several senolytic drugs are currently in clinical trials for a variety of age-related diseases, including cancer, fibrosis, and osteoarthritis. Another approach is to modulate the SASP itself. This can be achieved through anti-inflammatory drugs, or through targeted therapies that block the production or activity of specific SASP components. For instance, inhibiting interleukin-1 (IL-1), a pro-inflammatory cytokine that is often secreted by senescent cells, has shown promise in reducing inflammation and promoting tissue repair.

The emerging field of senotherapeutics, encompassing both senolytics and senomorphics (drugs that modulate the SASP), holds tremendous promise for promoting disease remission. However, significant challenges remain. One major challenge is the lack of specific biomarkers for identifying and tracking senescent cells in vivo. Without reliable biomarkers, it's difficult to assess the effectiveness of senotherapeutic interventions and to personalize treatment strategies. Another challenge is the potential for off-target effects. Senolytics, for example, may inadvertently kill healthy cells, leading to adverse side effects. Senomorphics, on the other hand, may have unintended consequences on other cellular processes. Careful preclinical and clinical testing is essential to ensure the safety and efficacy of senotherapeutic interventions. I think we are just starting to understand what senotherapeutics can do.

Moving forward, a deeper understanding of the molecular mechanisms that regulate cellular senescence and the SASP is crucial for developing more effective and targeted senotherapeutic strategies. This requires a multidisciplinary approach, integrating expertise in cell biology, immunology, pharmacology, and clinical medicine. Furthermore, it is crucial to understand the heterogeneity of senescent cells and the SASP in different disease contexts. Not all senescent cells are created equal, and the specific components of the SASP can vary depending on the type of cell, the stimulus that induced senescence, and the tissue microenvironment. Tailoring senotherapeutic interventions to the specific characteristics of senescent cells in each disease context may be necessary to maximize therapeutic efficacy and minimize adverse side effects. In conclusion, cellular senescence represents a critical and intricate factor in the pursuit of lasting disease remission. Understanding its multifaceted role, both beneficial and detrimental, and developing targeted strategies to manipulate it will be crucial for paving new avenues towards more effective and durable disease control. It is a field ripe with opportunity and challenge, demanding continued research and innovation to fully unlock its therapeutic potential.

3 Chapter 3: Immunotherapy's Role in Remission

The immune system, a complex and multifaceted network, stands as our primary defense against disease. For decades, researchers have sought ways to harness this power to not just manage illnesses, but to eradicate them entirely – to achieve true remission. Immunotherapy represents a paradigm shift, moving away from simply alleviating symptoms to actively engaging the body's own defenses. The beauty of this approach lies in its specificity; when properly directed, the immune system can target diseased cells with remarkable precision, minimizing collateral damage to healthy tissues.

Checkpoint inhibitors, one of the most significant breakthroughs in recent years, operate on a simple yet profound principle. Immune cells, specifically T cells, possess "checkpoints" – molecular brakes that prevent them from attacking healthy cells. Cancer cells, however, often exploit these checkpoints to evade immune detection. Drugs like pembrolizumab and nivolumab block these checkpoints, effectively releasing the brakes and unleashing the T cells to target and destroy cancer cells. The success of checkpoint inhibitors across various cancers, including melanoma, lung cancer, and Hodgkin lymphoma, has been nothing short of revolutionary, demonstrating the potential to induce durable remissions in patients who previously had limited options. This success has spurred intense research into identifying new checkpoint targets and developing even more effective inhibitors. However, it's crucial to acknowledge that checkpoint inhibitors are not without their challenges. Immune-related adverse events (irAEs), ranging from mild skin rashes to severe autoimmune reactions, can occur as a result of the immune system attacking healthy tissues. Careful monitoring and management of irAEs are essential to ensure patient safety and maximize the benefits of this powerful therapy.

Chimeric Antigen Receptor (CAR) T-cell therapy takes a different, highly personalized approach. In this process, a patient's own T cells are extracted and genetically modified to express a CAR, a synthetic receptor that specifically recognizes a protein found on the surface of cancer cells. These engineered CAR T cells are then infused back into the patient, where they can seek out and destroy cancer cells with remarkable efficiency. CAR T-cell therapy has shown dramatic success in treating certain blood cancers, particularly relapsed or refractory B-cell lymphomas and acute lymphoblastic leukemia (ALL) in children and young adults. The remission rates achieved with CAR T-cell therapy in these patient populations are often unprecedented, offering hope to those who have failed conventional treatments. However, CAR T-cell therapy is a complex and expensive procedure, and it is not without its risks. Cytokine release syndrome (CRS), a potentially life-threatening inflammatory response, is a common side effect. Neurotoxicity, affecting the nervous system, can also occur. Careful patient selection, meticulous monitoring, and prompt management of these complications are crucial for ensuring the safety and efficacy of CAR T-cell therapy.

The future of immunotherapy lies in personalization. Recognizing that each patient's disease is unique, researchers are developing strategies to tailor immunotherapies to individual characteristics. This includes analyzing the specific mutations within a patient's tumor, identifying the immune cells that are most likely to respond to therapy, and designing personalized vaccines that target tumor-specific antigens. Neoantigen vaccines, for example, are designed to target unique mutations found only in a patient's cancer cells. By training the immune system to recognize these neoantigens, these vaccines can elicit a highly specific and effective anti-tumor response. Furthermore, combination therapies are being explored to enhance the effectiveness of immunotherapy. Combining checkpoint inhibitors with other immunotherapeutic agents, targeted therapies, or even conventional chemotherapy, can often overcome resistance mechanisms and achieve deeper and more durable remissions. The development of biomarkers to predict which patients are most likely to respond to specific immunotherapies is also a major area of research. By identifying predictive biomarkers, clinicians can select the most appropriate treatment strategy for each patient, minimizing unnecessary side effects and maximizing the chances of success.

I believe that one of the most exciting frontiers in immuno-oncology is the development of therapies that target the tumor microenvironment. The tumor microenvironment, the complex ecosystem surrounding a tumor, plays a critical role in tumor growth, survival, and metastasis. It includes blood vessels, immune cells, fibroblasts, and other components that can either promote or suppress tumor progression. By targeting the tumor microenvironment, we can disrupt the support system that cancer cells rely on, making them more vulnerable to immunotherapy. I remember attending a conference where a researcher presented data on a novel therapy that targeted tumor-associated macrophages (TAMs), a type of immune cell that can promote tumor growth. The results were striking: the therapy not only reduced the number of TAMs in the tumor microenvironment but also enhanced the effectiveness of checkpoint inhibitors. This is just one example of how targeting the tumor microenvironment can improve the outcomes of immunotherapy. The quest for remission is a relentless one, demanding continuous innovation and a deep understanding of the intricate interplay between the immune system and disease. Immunotherapy, with its remarkable ability to harness the power of the body's own defenses, stands as a beacon of hope in this endeavor. As we continue to unravel the complexities of the immune system and refine our immunotherapeutic strategies, the dream of achieving durable remissions for an ever-growing number of patients is becoming increasingly within reach.

3.1 Harnessing the Immune System

Our immune system, a marvel of biological engineering, stands as a vigilant protector against a myriad of threats, from microscopic invaders to rogue cells within our own bodies. In the context of disease remission, particularly in areas like oncology and autoimmune disorders, understanding and harnessing the power of our immune defenses is paramount. This isn't merely about boosting immunity in a generic sense; it's about strategically directing the immune system to specifically target and eliminate the source of the disease, creating an environment where remission becomes not just possible, but sustainable. The journey towards utilizing the immune system effectively begins with recognizing its complexity and the multiple layers of regulation that govern its activity.

The immune system is not a single entity; rather, it is a complex network of cells, tissues, and organs that work in harmony to defend the body. It comprises two main arms: the innate and the adaptive immune systems. The innate immune system provides the first line of defense, offering a rapid but non-specific response to pathogens. Cells like macrophages and natural killer (NK) cells are key players, engulfing invaders and releasing inflammatory signals to recruit other immune cells. On the other hand, the adaptive immune system provides a more targeted and long-lasting immunity. T cells and B cells are the central components of this system, recognizing specific antigens (molecules on the surface of pathogens or diseased cells) and launching a tailored attack. T cells can directly kill infected cells or activate other immune cells, while B cells produce antibodies that neutralize pathogens and mark them for destruction. Understanding these fundamental components is essential for developing effective immunotherapeutic strategies. It's a ballet of biological processes, each with its specific cue and choreographed movement, working to maintain the balance of our internal world. If we are to conduct it, we must understand it, like any piece of music we want to play.

Now, let's explore how we can leverage this intricate system to achieve disease remission. One of the most promising approaches involves checkpoint inhibitors. These drugs work by blocking proteins, called checkpoints, that prevent T cells from attacking cancer cells. Imagine T cells as soldiers ready for battle, but held back by signals telling them to stand down. Checkpoint inhibitors release these brakes, allowing T cells to unleash their cytotoxic power against the tumor. Several checkpoint inhibitors, such as anti-PD-1 and anti-CTLA-4 antibodies, have shown remarkable success in treating various cancers, including melanoma, lung cancer, and Hodgkin lymphoma. For instance, patients with advanced melanoma who were once given a dismal prognosis are now experiencing long-term remission thanks to these therapies. However, checkpoint inhibitors are not without their limitations. They can cause immune-related adverse events, as the unleashed T cells may also attack healthy tissues. Careful patient selection and monitoring are crucial to minimize these side effects. Moreover, not all patients respond to checkpoint inhibitors, highlighting the need for predictive biomarkers to identify those most likely to benefit. It's a balancing act, fine-tuning the immune response to attack the disease without causing excessive harm to the body.

Moving beyond checkpoint inhibitors, CAR T-cell therapy represents another groundbreaking approach. This involves genetically engineering a patient's own T cells to express a chimeric antigen receptor (CAR) that recognizes a specific antigen on cancer cells. The engineered T cells are then infused back into the patient, where they can selectively target and destroy cancer cells expressing the target antigen. CAR T-cell therapy has shown remarkable success in treating certain blood cancers, particularly B-cell lymphomas and acute lymphoblastic leukemia. In some cases, patients who had relapsed after multiple lines of chemotherapy have achieved complete remission with CAR T-cell therapy. The process is complex and personalized, involving multiple steps from collecting the patient's T cells to manufacturing the CAR T cells and administering them back to the patient. While CAR T-cell therapy has revolutionized the treatment of certain cancers, it is also associated with potential toxicities, such as cytokine release syndrome (CRS) and neurotoxicity. CRS is caused by the massive release of cytokines from activated T cells, leading to systemic inflammation. Careful management of these toxicities is essential to ensure patient safety. Furthermore, CAR T-cell therapy is currently limited to a relatively small number of cancer types, and efforts are underway to expand its application to other solid tumors.

Personalized immunotherapy takes the concept of tailoring treatment to the individual patient to the next level. It involves analyzing a patient's unique immune profile and developing customized immunotherapeutic strategies based on their specific needs. This may include combining different immunotherapies, such as checkpoint inhibitors and vaccines, or designing personalized cancer vaccines that target specific antigens expressed by the patient's tumor. Advances in genomics and proteomics are enabling us to identify these unique antigens and develop highly targeted therapies. For example, neoantigens, which are tumor-specific antigens arising from mutations in cancer cells, can be used to create personalized cancer vaccines that stimulate the immune system to attack the tumor. The promise of personalized immunotherapy lies in its ability to overcome the limitations of one-size-fits-all approaches and deliver more effective and less toxic treatments. It requires a deep understanding of the patient's immune system, the tumor microenvironment, and the interplay between the two.

The future of immuno-oncology is brimming with possibilities. Combination therapies, where different immunotherapeutic agents are combined with each other or with other cancer treatments, such as chemotherapy or radiation therapy, are showing promising results. These combinations can overcome resistance mechanisms and enhance the effectiveness of immunotherapy. Another area of active research is the development of novel targets for immunotherapy. While PD-1 and CTLA-4 have been successful targets, there are many other immune checkpoints and stimulatory molecules that can be modulated to enhance the immune response against cancer. Furthermore, researchers are exploring new ways to deliver immunotherapies, such as using nanoparticles to target immune cells or engineering viruses to selectively infect and kill cancer cells. The convergence of immunology, genomics, and nanotechnology is paving the way for innovative and transformative approaches to disease remission. We stand on the cusp of a new era, where the immune system can be harnessed to conquer diseases that were once considered incurable. This requires a collaborative effort from scientists, clinicians, and patients, working together to unlock the full potential of immunotherapy.

In conclusion, harnessing the immune system represents a powerful strategy for achieving disease remission. From checkpoint inhibitors to CAR T-cell therapy and personalized immunotherapy, we have witnessed remarkable progress in recent years. While challenges remain, the future of immuno-oncology is bright, with ongoing research promising to deliver even more effective and less toxic treatments. As we continue to unravel the complexities of the immune system, we move closer to a world where disease remission becomes a reality for more patients, leading to longer, healthier lives. And I truly think, if we continue to progress in this direction, we can bring great things to patients.

3.2 Checkpoint Inhibitors and Remission

Immune checkpoints are essentially brakes on the immune system, preventing it from overreacting and attacking healthy tissues. However, in the context of cancer, this regulatory mechanism can be exploited by tumor cells to evade immune destruction. They are molecules on immune cells, like T cells, that need to be either activated or inactivated to start or stop an immune response. These checkpoints are vital for preventing autoimmunity, but cancer cells can hijack them to suppress the immune system and avoid being killed. Enter checkpoint inhibitors – drugs designed to release these brakes, unleashing the full power of the immune system to recognize and destroy cancer cells. By blocking these checkpoints, the immune system is reactivated, allowing T cells to effectively target and eliminate tumor cells, potentially leading to significant tumor regression and, in some cases, even remission.

The journey of checkpoint inhibitors from the laboratory to the clinic is a remarkable story of scientific discovery and clinical innovation. Early research focused on understanding the fundamental mechanisms of T cell activation and regulation. Scientists identified key checkpoint molecules, such as CTLA-4 and PD-1, and elucidated their roles in suppressing immune responses. The pivotal breakthrough came with the development of monoclonal antibodies that could specifically block these checkpoint molecules, effectively unleashing the anti-tumor activity of T cells. The initial clinical trials with checkpoint inhibitors yielded astonishing results, demonstrating unprecedented response rates and durable remissions in patients with advanced cancers, such as melanoma, that had previously been considered incurable. These findings revolutionized cancer treatment and paved the way for the widespread adoption of checkpoint inhibitors across a wide range of malignancies.

CTLA-4 was one of the first checkpoint molecules to be targeted therapeutically. It primarily acts in the early stages of T cell activation, dampening the initial immune response. Ipilimumab, an anti-CTLA-4 antibody, was the first checkpoint inhibitor to gain FDA approval for the treatment of metastatic melanoma. While ipilimumab can induce durable remissions in some patients, it is also associated with significant immune-related adverse events (irAEs) due to its broad effect on the immune system. Therefore, careful patient selection and management of irAEs are crucial for optimizing treatment outcomes.

PD-1 and its ligand PD-L1 represent another critical checkpoint pathway. PD-1 is expressed on activated T cells, while PD-L1 is frequently expressed on tumor cells and other immune cells in the tumor microenvironment. The interaction between PD-1 and PD-L1 inhibits T cell activity and allows tumor cells to evade immune destruction. Anti-PD-1 antibodies, such as nivolumab and pembrolizumab, and anti-PD-L1 antibodies, such as atezolizumab and durvalumab, have demonstrated remarkable efficacy across a wide range of cancers, including melanoma, lung cancer, kidney cancer, bladder cancer, and Hodgkin lymphoma. These agents generally have a more favorable safety profile compared to anti-CTLA-4 antibodies, although irAEs can still occur.

While checkpoint inhibitors have revolutionized cancer treatment, they are not without their challenges. One major challenge is that not all patients respond to checkpoint inhibitor therapy. Biomarkers, such as PD-L1 expression, tumor mutational burden (TMB), and microsatellite instability (MSI), can help predict response to checkpoint inhibitors, but they are not perfect predictors. Research is ongoing to identify novel biomarkers that can better predict response and guide treatment decisions. Another challenge is the development of resistance to checkpoint inhibitors. Tumor cells can develop various mechanisms to evade immune destruction, such as downregulating PD-L1 expression, mutating checkpoint pathways, or recruiting immunosuppressive cells to the tumor microenvironment. Strategies to overcome resistance include combining checkpoint inhibitors with other therapies, such as chemotherapy, targeted therapy, or radiation therapy, and developing novel immunotherapeutic agents that target different immune pathways. Managing immune-related adverse events (irAEs) is also a critical aspect of checkpoint inhibitor therapy. IrAEs can affect virtually any organ system and range in severity from mild to life-threatening. Early recognition and prompt management of irAEs are essential to minimize morbidity and maintain treatment efficacy.

The future of checkpoint inhibitor therapy is bright. Ongoing research is focused on developing novel checkpoint inhibitors that target different immune pathways, identifying predictive biomarkers to guide treatment decisions, and developing strategies to overcome resistance. Combination therapies involving checkpoint inhibitors and other immunotherapeutic agents, such as CAR T-cell therapy and oncolytic viruses, are also being explored. These advances hold the promise of further improving outcomes for patients with cancer and expanding the reach of checkpoint inhibitor therapy to even more malignancies. I believe that one day, we will see checkpoint inhibitors play a significant role in achieving long-term remission for many more cancer patients. In some cases, it might even eradicate the disease entirely. We have already seen such cases reported over the last years, and this is the reason why I firmly believe that with even more research we can provide a better future for every patient and their families.

3.3 CAR T-Cell Therapy Advances

Chimeric antigen receptor (CAR) T-cell therapy has revolutionized the treatment of certain cancers, particularly hematologic malignancies, offering the potential for durable remissions in patients who have exhausted other treatment options. The fundamental principle of CAR T-cell therapy is to engineer a patient's own T cells to recognize and attack cancer cells expressing a specific antigen. This involves collecting T cells from the patient's blood (a process called leukapheresis), genetically modifying them in a laboratory to express a CAR targeting a specific antigen found on cancer cells, expanding the modified T cells in culture, and then infusing them back into the patient.

The CAR itself is a synthetic receptor designed to redirect T-cell specificity. It typically consists of an extracellular antigen-binding domain, often derived from a single-chain variable fragment (scFv) of an antibody, linked to intracellular signaling domains that activate the T cell upon antigen recognition. First-generation CARs contained only a single intracellular signaling domain, typically CD3, and demonstrated limited efficacy. Second-generation CARs incorporated an additional costimulatory domain, such as CD28 or 4-1BB, to enhance T-cell activation, proliferation, and persistence. Third-generation CARs added a second costimulatory domain, aiming to further improve T-cell function. However, clinical experience has shown that second-generation CARs generally provide a good balance of efficacy and safety. Newer generations are in development.

While CD19-directed CAR T-cell therapy has shown remarkable success in treating relapsed/refractory B-cell lymphomas and acute lymphoblastic leukemia (ALL), challenges remain. One significant obstacle is the occurrence of cytokine release syndrome (CRS), a systemic inflammatory response triggered by the activation and proliferation of CAR T cells. CRS can manifest with a range of symptoms, from fever and fatigue to life-threatening organ dysfunction. Management strategies for CRS include supportive care, such as fluids and vasopressors, as well as immunosuppressive agents like tocilizumab, an IL-6 receptor antagonist, and corticosteroids. Another notable adverse event is immune effector cell-associated neurotoxicity syndrome (ICANS), which can cause neurological symptoms ranging from confusion and tremor to seizures and coma. The mechanisms underlying ICANS are not fully understood, but it is thought to involve cytokine-mediated inflammation and disruption of the blood-brain barrier. Management of ICANS also involves supportive care and immunosuppression.

Strategies to mitigate the toxicity of CAR T-cell therapy are actively being explored. One approach is to develop CARs with improved safety profiles, such as those incorporating "suicide genes" that can be activated to eliminate CAR T cells if severe toxicity occurs. Another strategy is to optimize the CAR T-cell manufacturing process to generate products with more predictable and controlled activation properties. Furthermore, researchers are investigating the use of prophylactic immunosuppression to prevent or reduce the severity of CRS and ICANS. In addition to toxicity management, efforts are underway to enhance the efficacy of CAR T-cell therapy. One area of focus is to overcome resistance mechanisms that can limit the durability of response. These mechanisms can include antigen escape, where cancer cells downregulate or lose expression of the target antigen, and T-cell exhaustion, where CAR T cells become functionally impaired over time. Strategies to address antigen escape include developing CAR T cells targeting multiple antigens or using bispecific CARs that recognize two different antigens on the same cancer cell. To overcome T-cell exhaustion, researchers are exploring approaches such as incorporating checkpoint inhibitors into the CAR T-cell product or genetically modifying CAR T cells to enhance their persistence and effector function.

Beyond B-cell malignancies, CAR T-cell therapy is being investigated for a wide range of other cancers, including solid tumors. However, targeting solid tumors with CAR T cells presents unique challenges. Solid tumors often exhibit a heterogeneous expression of target antigens, and the tumor microenvironment can be immunosuppressive, hindering CAR T-cell infiltration and activity. Moreover, identifying tumor-specific antigens that are not expressed on normal tissues is crucial to avoid on-target, off-tumor toxicity. Despite these challenges, significant progress is being made in developing CAR T-cell therapies for solid tumors. Researchers are exploring strategies to enhance CAR T-cell trafficking to the tumor site, overcome immunosuppression, and improve target antigen selection.

The field of CAR T-cell therapy is rapidly evolving, with ongoing research focused on improving efficacy, reducing toxicity, and expanding the application of this powerful technology to a wider range of cancers. As we delve deeper into understanding the complexities of the immune system and the mechanisms of cancer resistance, we can anticipate further advances in CAR T-cell therapy that will ultimately lead to more durable remissions and improved outcomes for patients with life-threatening malignancies. Innovations are happening at the cellular level to enhance CAR T-cell performance. We are also seeing changes in manufacturing to help more patients receive this important therapy.

3.4 Personalized Immunotherapy Strategies

The concept of personalized immunotherapy pivots on the profound understanding that each individual's immune system and disease profile are unique. What works effectively for one patient may yield minimal or even adverse results in another. Therefore, a one-size-fits-all approach to immunotherapy is often inadequate, particularly when striving for lasting disease remission. Instead, personalized strategies tailor treatment to the specific characteristics of the patient, their disease, and their immune response, maximizing the potential for effective and durable outcomes. Achieving this level of precision requires a multifaceted approach encompassing advanced diagnostics, sophisticated data analysis, and innovative therapeutic design.

The initial step in crafting a personalized immunotherapy strategy involves a comprehensive assessment of the patient's disease. This extends far beyond traditional diagnostic methods and incorporates advanced techniques like genomic sequencing, proteomic analysis, and metabolomic profiling. Genomic sequencing identifies specific genetic mutations within the diseased cells that may serve as therapeutic targets or predict response to certain immunotherapies. For instance, identifying specific mutations in genes like EGFR or ALK in lung cancer patients can guide the selection of targeted therapies that enhance the effectiveness of immunotherapy. Proteomic analysis, on the other hand, examines the expression levels of proteins within the diseased cells and the surrounding microenvironment. This provides a more dynamic picture of the disease state and can reveal potential biomarkers that predict response or resistance to immunotherapy. Metabolomic profiling analyzes the metabolic products produced by the diseased cells, offering insights into their metabolic pathways and vulnerabilities. By combining these advanced diagnostic approaches, clinicians can gain a holistic understanding of the patient's disease, paving the way for a truly personalized treatment strategy.

Beyond characterizing the disease itself, a thorough assessment of the patient's immune system is equally critical. This involves evaluating the composition and function of various immune cell populations, such as T cells, B cells, and natural killer (NK) cells. Flow cytometry is a powerful technique used to identify and quantify these immune cell populations in the patient's blood or tissue samples. By analyzing the expression of specific surface markers on these cells, clinicians can determine their activation state, functionality, and potential to mount an effective immune response against the disease. In addition to flow cytometry, functional assays can assess the ability of these immune cells to kill diseased cells, produce cytokines, and proliferate in response to stimulation. These assays provide valuable information about the overall health and responsiveness of the patient's immune system. Furthermore, analyzing the patient's cytokine profile can reveal underlying immune dysregulation or chronic inflammation that may impact the effectiveness of immunotherapy. By understanding the patient's immune landscape, clinicians can tailor immunotherapy strategies to boost specific immune functions and overcome immune suppression.

Harnessing the power of neoantigens represents a cutting-edge approach in personalized immunotherapy. Neoantigens are unique protein fragments present on the surface of diseased cells that arise from genetic mutations specific to that individual's disease. Because these neoantigens are not found on normal cells, they represent highly specific targets for the immune system. Identifying and targeting neoantigens can trigger a potent and selective immune response against the disease, minimizing the risk of off-target effects. The process of identifying neoantigens involves sophisticated bioinformatics analysis of the patient's genomic sequencing data. Algorithms are used to predict which mutations are likely to generate neoantigens that can be recognized by the immune system. Once potential neoantigens are identified, they can be synthesized and used to stimulate the patient's immune cells in vitro. This allows clinicians to assess whether the patient's immune system can mount a response against these neoantigens. If a strong immune response is observed, the neoantigens can be incorporated into personalized vaccines or used to engineer T cells that specifically target the disease. This approach holds immense promise for achieving durable disease remission by directing the immune system to attack the unique fingerprint of the patient's disease.

The gut microbiome, a complex ecosystem of bacteria, viruses, fungi, and other microorganisms residing in the digestive tract, has emerged as a critical factor influencing the efficacy of immunotherapy. Emerging evidence suggests that the composition and diversity of the gut microbiome can significantly impact the patient's immune response and their likelihood of responding to immunotherapy. Certain gut bacteria have been shown to enhance the activity of immune cells, while others can suppress the immune system. Manipulating the gut microbiome through dietary interventions, fecal microbiota transplantation (FMT), or the use of probiotics may improve the effectiveness of immunotherapy. Dietary interventions involve modifying the patient's diet to promote the growth of beneficial bacteria and reduce the abundance of harmful bacteria. FMT involves transferring fecal material from a healthy donor to the patient's gut, with the goal of restoring a healthy microbiome. Probiotics are live microorganisms that, when administered in adequate amounts, confer a health benefit on the host. Clinical trials are underway to investigate the impact of these microbiome-modulating strategies on immunotherapy outcomes. By optimizing the gut microbiome, clinicians can potentially enhance the patient's immune response and improve their chances of achieving durable disease remission.

Combining different immunotherapeutic modalities can often lead to synergistic effects and improved outcomes compared to single-agent approaches. For example, combining checkpoint inhibitors with adoptive cell therapies or oncolytic viruses can enhance the immune response and overcome resistance mechanisms. Checkpoint inhibitors work by blocking proteins that suppress the immune system, allowing immune cells to more effectively attack diseased cells. Adoptive cell therapies, such as CAR T-cell therapy, involve engineering the patient's own immune cells to specifically target the disease. Oncolytic viruses are genetically modified viruses that selectively infect and kill diseased cells, while also stimulating an immune response. By combining these different approaches, clinicians can target multiple pathways and achieve a more comprehensive and durable immune response. However, it is important to carefully consider the potential for overlapping toxicities when combining immunotherapies. Close monitoring of patients and proactive management of side effects are essential to ensure patient safety. The optimal combination of immunotherapies will depend on the specific characteristics of the patient, their disease, and their immune response.

3.5 Future Directions in Immuno-Oncology

The journey of immuno-oncology is far from over; it's a rapidly evolving landscape teeming with possibilities. We've witnessed the transformative power of checkpoint inhibitors and CAR T-cell therapy, but these are just the initial forays. The future beckons with promises of more refined, personalized, and effective strategies. One promising avenue lies in the development of combinatorial immunotherapies. Instead of relying on a single agent, researchers are exploring synergistic combinations that can overcome resistance mechanisms and enhance anti-tumor responses. For instance, combining checkpoint inhibitors with oncolytic viruses, which selectively infect and destroy cancer cells while stimulating an immune response, may provide a potent one-two punch. Furthermore, innovative combinations could involve targeting multiple immune checkpoints simultaneously or combining immunotherapy with conventional therapies like chemotherapy or radiation. The key lies in understanding the complex interplay between different immune pathways and identifying the optimal combinations to maximize efficacy while minimizing toxicity. Beyond combinations, there's a growing focus on personalized neoantigen-based therapies. Neoantigens are unique mutations found in cancer cells that aren't present in normal cells, making them ideal targets for the immune system. By identifying these neoantigens in individual patients, scientists can create personalized vaccines or T-cell therapies that specifically target their tumors. This approach holds immense potential for overcoming tumor heterogeneity and preventing immune evasion. However, the development of neoantigen-based therapies is not without its challenges. Identifying relevant neoantigens can be complex and time-consuming, and the manufacturing of personalized therapies is often expensive and logistically demanding. Nevertheless, ongoing advancements in genomics, bioinformatics, and manufacturing technologies are paving the way for more efficient and cost-effective neoantigen-based approaches.

Another exciting area of research is focused on modulating the tumor microenvironment (TME) to enhance immune cell infiltration and activity. The TME is a complex ecosystem surrounding the tumor, comprising immune cells, blood vessels, and stromal cells. Often, the TME is immunosuppressive, preventing immune cells from effectively attacking the tumor. Strategies aimed at remodeling the TME include targeting immunosuppressive cells like myeloid-derived suppressor cells (MDSCs) and regulatory T cells (Tregs), which can dampen the immune response. Researchers are also exploring ways to enhance the recruitment and activation of cytotoxic T cells and natural killer (NK) cells within the TME. Furthermore, manipulating the tumor vasculature to improve drug delivery and immune cell infiltration is another promising approach. By transforming the TME from an immunosuppressive to an immunostimulatory environment, we can unlock the full potential of immunotherapies.

The adoptive cell therapy landscape is also expanding beyond CAR T-cells. While CAR T-cell therapy has shown remarkable success in hematological malignancies, its efficacy in solid tumors has been limited. Researchers are exploring alternative adoptive cell therapies, such as T-cell receptor (TCR) engineered T cells, which can recognize a broader range of tumor-associated antigens, and tumor-infiltrating lymphocytes (TILs), which are naturally occurring immune cells that have already infiltrated the tumor. Furthermore, advancements in gene editing technologies, such as CRISPR-Cas9, are enabling the creation of more sophisticated and potent adoptive cell therapies with enhanced targeting capabilities and reduced off-target effects. The future of adoptive cell therapy lies in identifying the optimal cell type, engineering strategy, and delivery method to maximize efficacy and safety in a wider range of cancers.

Furthermore, oncolytic viruses (OVs) represent a particularly interesting area of development. They can selectively infect and kill cancer cells, but their impact goes far beyond direct destruction. As OVs replicate within tumor cells, they trigger an inflammatory response, alerting the immune system to the presence of the tumor. This, in turn, can stimulate a broader, more durable anti-tumor immune response. Moreover, OVs can be engineered to express therapeutic genes, such as cytokines or checkpoint inhibitors, further enhancing their anti-tumor activity. Clinical trials are underway to evaluate the safety and efficacy of OVs in various cancers, both as monotherapy and in combination with other immunotherapies. OVs hold the potential to transform the treatment landscape, particularly for cancers that are resistant to other forms of immunotherapy.

As we move forward, it's crucial to remember that the path to successful immunotherapy is not always linear. Resistance to immunotherapy remains a significant challenge. Tumors can develop various mechanisms to evade the immune system, such as downregulating target antigens, upregulating inhibitory molecules, or altering the tumor microenvironment. Overcoming resistance requires a deeper understanding of these mechanisms and the development of strategies to counteract them. This might involve combining different immunotherapies, targeting multiple pathways simultaneously, or developing novel agents that specifically address resistance mechanisms.

Finally, biomarkers play a pivotal role in predicting response to immunotherapy and guiding treatment decisions. Currently, PD-L1 expression is a commonly used biomarker for checkpoint inhibitor therapy, but it is not always a reliable predictor of response. Researchers are actively searching for more accurate and predictive biomarkers, such as tumor mutational burden (TMB), microsatellite instability (MSI), and gene expression signatures. These biomarkers can help identify patients who are most likely to benefit from immunotherapy and guide the selection of the most appropriate treatment strategy. The development of more sophisticated and personalized biomarker approaches is essential for optimizing immunotherapy outcomes and ensuring that patients receive the most effective treatment possible. The future of disease treatment hinges on the integration of all these advances, creating a tapestry of therapeutic options tailored to each individual's unique disease profile.

4 Chapter 4: Targeted Therapies and Precision Medicine

The promise of precision medicine lies in its ability to tailor treatments to the individual characteristics of a patient's disease, not just the disease itself. This approach hinges on identifying specific molecular alterations that drive disease progression, allowing clinicians to select therapies that target these vulnerabilities directly. Unlike traditional "one-size-fits-all" treatments, targeted therapies are designed to interfere with specific molecules or pathways involved in tumor growth, proliferation, or survival. This specificity translates into potentially higher efficacy and fewer off-target effects, which can lead to a better quality of life during treatment and a more durable remission.

Genomic profiling forms the cornerstone of targeted therapy. Techniques such as next-generation sequencing (NGS) allow us to analyze the entire genome, or specific regions of interest, to identify mutations, amplifications, deletions, and other genomic aberrations that may be driving the disease. For example, in lung cancer, identifying mutations in genes like EGFR, ALK, or ROS1 allows physicians to prescribe specific tyrosine kinase inhibitors (TKIs) that target these altered proteins, leading to significant tumor shrinkage and improved survival rates. Similarly, in melanoma, the presence of a BRAF mutation can be targeted with BRAF inhibitors, often in combination with MEK inhibitors, leading to rapid and significant clinical responses. The information gleaned from genomic profiling is not limited to identifying drug targets; it can also be used to predict prognosis, monitor treatment response, and identify potential mechanisms of resistance. In essence, comprehensive genomic profiling provides a detailed blueprint of the disease, guiding treatment decisions and maximizing the likelihood of achieving remission.

Small molecule inhibitors represent a significant class of targeted therapies that have revolutionized the treatment of various diseases. These inhibitors are designed to bind to specific protein targets, such as kinases, enzymes, or receptors, and block their activity. Their relatively small size allows them to readily enter cells and interact with intracellular targets. One of the earliest and most celebrated success stories of small molecule inhibitors is imatinib, used in the treatment of chronic myeloid leukemia (CML). Imatinib specifically inhibits the BCR-ABL tyrosine kinase, which is constitutively active in CML cells, leading to uncontrolled proliferation. Before imatinib, CML was a deadly disease with limited treatment options. Today, thanks to imatinib and other similar inhibitors, many patients with CML can achieve long-term remission and live normal lives. Another example is the use of EGFR inhibitors in non-small cell lung cancer (NSCLC) harboring EGFR mutations. These inhibitors have demonstrated remarkable efficacy in shrinking tumors and extending survival in patients with EGFR-mutant NSCLC. Other success stories include the use of BRAF and MEK inhibitors in melanoma, ALK inhibitors in ALK-positive NSCLC, and PARP inhibitors in ovarian cancer with BRCA mutations. These examples highlight the power of small molecule inhibitors to target specific vulnerabilities in cancer cells and induce remission.

However, the success of targeted therapies is often limited by the emergence of resistance. Cancer cells are masters of adaptation, and they can develop various mechanisms to evade the effects of targeted drugs. These mechanisms can include acquiring new mutations in the target protein that prevent the drug from binding, activating alternative signaling pathways that bypass the inhibited target, or increasing expression of drug efflux pumps that pump the drug out of the cell. Overcoming resistance is a major challenge in targeted therapy, and researchers are actively exploring various strategies to address this issue. One approach is to develop second-generation inhibitors that can overcome resistance mutations. For example, several second-generation EGFR inhibitors have been developed to target EGFR mutations that confer resistance to first-generation inhibitors. Another strategy is to combine targeted therapies with other treatments, such as chemotherapy, immunotherapy, or radiation therapy, to attack cancer cells from multiple angles and prevent the development of resistance. A third approach is to target resistance mechanisms directly. For example, inhibitors of drug efflux pumps can be used to increase the intracellular concentration of targeted drugs and overcome resistance. Furthermore, understanding the specific mechanisms of resistance in each patient through repeated genomic profiling can guide the selection of alternative therapies or combination strategies. By continuously monitoring the genomic landscape of the disease and adapting treatment accordingly, we can improve the durability of remission and prevent relapse.

The application of targeted therapies extends beyond oncology to other diseases as well. In autoimmune diseases, for example, targeted therapies are being developed to inhibit specific immune cells or cytokines that contribute to inflammation and tissue damage. In infectious diseases, targeted therapies are being explored to inhibit viral replication or bacterial virulence factors. The principles of precision medicine—identifying specific molecular targets and developing therapies that selectively interfere with them—are applicable to a wide range of diseases, offering the potential to revolutionize treatment and improve patient outcomes across the board.

I firmly believe the future of disease management lies in the integration of genomic profiling, targeted therapies, and personalized medicine. By understanding the unique molecular characteristics of each patient's disease, we can select the most appropriate treatments, monitor treatment response, and adapt our strategies as needed to overcome resistance and achieve durable remission. This approach requires a multidisciplinary team of experts, including physicians, scientists, genetic counselors, and bioinformaticians, working together to translate genomic data into clinical decisions. Furthermore, it requires investment in research and development to discover new targets, develop novel therapies, and improve our understanding of resistance mechanisms. While challenges remain, the promise of targeted therapies and precision medicine is undeniable. By continuing to advance our knowledge and refine our approaches, we can pave the way for a future where diseases are treated with precision and patients can achieve lasting remission and improved quality of life.

4.1 Genomic Profiling for Targeted Approaches

The advent of targeted therapies has revolutionized disease management, shifting the paradigm from generalized treatments to personalized strategies tailored to an individual's unique genetic makeup. At the heart of this transformative approach lies genomic profiling, a powerful tool that deciphers the genetic code of a patient's cells, revealing actionable insights that can guide treatment decisions and enhance the likelihood of remission. This chapter will delve into the fundamentals of genomic profiling, exploring its various methodologies, clinical applications, and its pivotal role in paving new avenues for disease remission.

Genomic profiling, in its essence, is the process of analyzing an individual's DNA or RNA to identify genetic variations, mutations, or other molecular markers that are associated with a particular disease. This information can then be used to understand the underlying mechanisms driving the disease, predict treatment response, and ultimately, select the most effective therapeutic strategy for each patient. There exists a wide array of techniques employed in genomic profiling, each with its own strengths and limitations. These include, but are not limited to, single-gene sequencing, which focuses on analyzing specific genes known to be involved in disease development; multi-gene panels, which simultaneously assess multiple genes related to a particular disease; whole-exome sequencing (WES), which examines the protein-coding regions of all genes in the genome; and whole-genome sequencing (WGS), which provides a comprehensive analysis of the entire genome. RNA sequencing (RNA-Seq) is also crucial as it measures gene expression levels, reflecting the activity of genes within a cell. Each method provides different levels of detail and is appropriate for different clinical scenarios, based on the complexity of the disease and the desired depth of analysis.

The clinical applications of genomic profiling are vast and continue to expand across various medical specialties. In oncology, genomic profiling has become an indispensable tool for guiding treatment decisions in various cancers. For instance, in lung cancer, identifying mutations in genes such as EGFR, ALK, and ROS1 can determine whether a patient is eligible for targeted therapies that specifically inhibit the activity of these mutated proteins. Similarly, in breast cancer, genomic profiling assays like Oncotype DX and MammaPrint can predict the likelihood of recurrence and help guide decisions about adjuvant chemotherapy. These tests analyze the expression of multiple genes to provide a personalized risk assessment and determine the potential benefit of chemotherapy. Beyond oncology, genomic profiling is also playing an increasingly important role in other fields of medicine. In cardiology, it can be used to identify individuals at risk for inherited cardiac conditions such as hypertrophic cardiomyopathy and long QT syndrome. In neurology, it can aid in the diagnosis of genetic disorders such as Huntington's disease and spinal muscular atrophy. In infectious diseases, genomic profiling can be used to track the spread of pathogens and identify drug-resistant strains.

Precision medicine, fueled by genomic profiling, tailors treatment to the individual, minimizing off-target effects and maximizing therapeutic efficacy. This approach contrasts sharply with traditional, one-size-fits-all treatments that often result in suboptimal outcomes and unnecessary side effects. In the realm of drug development, genomic profiling is helping to identify potential drug targets and stratify patients for clinical trials, increasing the likelihood of success and accelerating the development of new therapies. A crucial aspect of genomic profiling is the interpretation of the vast amount of data generated. This requires specialized expertise in bioinformatics and genetics, as well as access to comprehensive databases and analytical tools. The interpretation of genomic data should always be performed in the context of a patient's clinical history, physical examination findings, and other relevant laboratory results. It is also important to consider the limitations of genomic profiling, such as the possibility of false-positive or false-negative results, and the potential for incidental findings that may have uncertain clinical significance.

Overcoming resistance to targeted therapies is a major challenge in disease management. Genomic profiling can play a crucial role in identifying the mechanisms of resistance and guiding the selection of alternative therapies. For example, in patients with EGFR-mutated lung cancer who develop resistance to first-generation EGFR inhibitors, genomic profiling can identify the presence of a T790M mutation, which confers resistance to these drugs. This information can then be used to select a third-generation EGFR inhibitor, such as osimertinib, which is specifically designed to overcome the T790M mutation. The integration of genomic profiling into clinical practice also raises several ethical considerations. One important issue is the privacy and security of genomic data. It is crucial to ensure that genomic information is protected from unauthorized access and misuse.

Another ethical consideration is the potential for genetic discrimination, where individuals are discriminated against based on their genetic predispositions. To address these concerns, it is important to have robust policies and regulations in place to protect individuals' genetic rights.
Looking ahead, the future of genomic profiling holds immense promise. Advances in sequencing technologies are making genomic profiling faster, cheaper, and more accessible. The development of new analytical tools and databases is improving our ability to interpret genomic data and translate it into clinically actionable insights. The integration of genomic profiling with other omics technologies, such as proteomics and metabolomics, is providing a more comprehensive understanding of disease biology. As genomic profiling becomes more widely adopted, it is poised to transform the way we diagnose, treat, and prevent diseases, paving the way for a future where medicine is truly personalized and tailored to the unique needs of each individual. Indeed, this precision, guided by the insights gleaned from our own genetic blueprint, offers the best hope for achieving durable remission and improving the lives of countless individuals grappling with disease.

4.2 Small Molecule Inhibitors: Success Stories

Imagine a world where chronic myeloid leukemia (CML), once a death sentence, could be managed with a single daily pill. This isn't science fiction; it's the reality shaped by imatinib, a small molecule inhibitor that revolutionized CML treatment. Prior to imatinib's introduction, the primary treatment for CML was bone marrow transplantation, a risky and often debilitating procedure. Interferon-alpha offered another option, but its side effects were significant, and complete remission was rare. Then, in the late 1990s, came a glimmer of hope. Imatinib, designed to specifically target the BCR-ABL fusion protein – the driving force behind CML – entered clinical trials. The results were nothing short of astonishing. Patients who had failed other treatments experienced dramatic reductions in leukemic cells. Many achieved complete hematologic remission, meaning their blood counts returned to normal. This wasn't just about extending life; it was about restoring quality of life. People who had been confined to their homes due to fatigue and the constant threat of infection were now able to return to work, travel, and enjoy time with their families. Imatinib became a symbol of targeted therapy's potential, a testament to the power of designing drugs that selectively attack the molecular underpinnings of disease.

The success of imatinib paved the way for other small molecule inhibitors to enter the oncology landscape, each targeting specific cancer-driving mutations. Consider vemurafenib, a drug that targets the BRAF V600E mutation, commonly found in melanoma. Before vemurafenib, metastatic melanoma was notoriously difficult to treat, with limited therapeutic options and a grim prognosis. Chemotherapy offered marginal benefit, and the five-year survival rate was dismally low. Vemurafenib changed that paradigm. Patients with the BRAF V600E mutation who received vemurafenib experienced significant tumor shrinkage and improved survival. The drug's impact was so profound that it quickly became the standard of care for this subset of melanoma patients. However, the story didn't end there. Cancer cells are remarkably adaptable, and resistance to vemurafenib inevitably emerged. Researchers discovered that cancer cells could bypass the drug's effect by activating alternative signaling pathways. This led to the development of combination therapies that targeted multiple pathways simultaneously, delaying the onset of resistance and further improving patient outcomes. The vemurafenib story highlights both the remarkable potential and the inherent challenges of targeted therapy: while these drugs can achieve remarkable results, the development of resistance remains a constant concern.

Beyond oncology, small molecule inhibitors have also proven effective in treating autoimmune diseases. Tofacitinib, for example, is a Janus kinase (JAK) inhibitor approved for the treatment of rheumatoid arthritis (RA). RA is a chronic inflammatory disorder that causes pain, swelling, and stiffness in the joints. While traditional therapies like methotrexate can provide some relief, many patients fail to respond adequately or experience significant side effects. Tofacitinib offers an alternative approach by blocking the activity of JAK enzymes, which play a crucial role in signaling pathways involved in inflammation. Clinical trials have demonstrated that tofacitinib can significantly reduce RA symptoms and improve joint function. For many patients, this translates to a substantial improvement in their quality of life, allowing them to participate more fully in daily activities. The success of tofacitinib has spurred the development of other JAK inhibitors for various autoimmune conditions, expanding the therapeutic options for patients suffering from these debilitating diseases.

The journey from identifying a disease target to developing a successful small molecule inhibitor is a complex and lengthy process. It begins with basic research to understand the molecular mechanisms underlying the disease. Once a promising target is identified, researchers use a variety of techniques, including high-throughput screening and rational drug design, to identify molecules that can bind to and inhibit the target protein. These molecules then undergo extensive preclinical testing in cell cultures and animal models to assess their efficacy and safety. If the preclinical data are promising, the molecule can then proceed to clinical trials in humans. Clinical trials are conducted in three phases, each designed to evaluate different aspects of the drug, including its safety, efficacy, and optimal dosage. Only a small fraction of molecules that enter preclinical testing ultimately make it through all phases of clinical trials and are approved for use in patients. This rigorous process is essential to ensure that new drugs are both effective and safe. The development of each successful small molecule inhibitor represents a significant investment of time, resources, and scientific expertise.

One of the major challenges in developing small molecule inhibitors is ensuring that they are selective for their intended target. Many proteins share similar structural features, and a drug that binds to one protein may also bind to others, leading to unwanted side effects. Researchers use a variety of techniques to improve the selectivity of their drugs, including modifying the chemical structure of the molecule and optimizing its binding properties. Another challenge is overcoming drug resistance. As mentioned earlier, cancer cells and other disease-causing cells can develop resistance to targeted therapies by activating alternative signaling pathways or mutating the drug target. Researchers are constantly working to understand the mechanisms of resistance and to develop strategies to overcome them. These strategies include developing combination therapies that target multiple pathways simultaneously, designing drugs that are less susceptible to resistance, and using personalized medicine approaches to select the most effective treatment for each patient. Despite these challenges, the field of small molecule inhibitors continues to advance rapidly, driven by advances in our understanding of disease biology and by innovations in drug discovery technology.

As we look to the future, the potential of small molecule inhibitors remains immense. With ongoing advances in genomics, proteomics, and other fields, we are gaining a deeper understanding of the molecular complexities of disease. This knowledge is enabling us to identify new and more effective drug targets. Furthermore, advances in drug discovery technologies, such as artificial intelligence and machine learning, are accelerating the process of identifying and optimizing new drug candidates. These technologies can analyze vast amounts of data to predict which molecules are most likely to be effective and safe. The combination of these advances promises to usher in a new era of targeted therapies, offering the potential to treat a wide range of diseases with greater precision and efficacy. The legacy of imatinib and other successful small molecule inhibitors serves as an inspiration to researchers and clinicians alike, driving the ongoing quest to develop innovative therapies that can transform the lives of patients. By continuing to invest in basic research, drug discovery, and clinical trials, we can unlock the full potential of small molecule inhibitors and pave the way for a future where disease remission is a reality for more and more people.

4.3 Resistance Mechanisms and Overcoming Them

Resistance to targeted therapies represents a significant hurdle in achieving lasting disease remission. While initial responses to these drugs can be promising, the development of resistance often leads to disease recurrence, necessitating a deeper understanding of the underlying mechanisms and strategies to overcome them. One of the primary mechanisms of resistance involves alterations in the drug target itself. This can manifest as mutations that prevent the drug from binding effectively, conformational changes that reduce drug efficacy, or even upregulation of the target protein, overwhelming the drug's inhibitory capacity. For instance, in cancers treated with EGFR inhibitors, mutations in the EGFR kinase domain can render the drug ineffective by preventing its binding. Strategies to address this include developing second\item or third-generation inhibitors that are specifically designed to overcome these mutations. These newer drugs may have a different binding mode or increased affinity for the mutated target, allowing them to effectively inhibit the protein's activity despite the presence of resistance-conferring mutations.

Another prevalent mechanism involves the activation of bypass pathways. These are alternative signaling routes that can compensate for the inhibition of the primary target. When a targeted therapy blocks a specific pathway, cells may activate other pathways that can circumvent the block and maintain downstream signaling, effectively bypassing the intended therapeutic effect. For example, in certain cancers, inhibition of the PI3K/AKT/mTOR pathway can lead to the activation of the MAPK pathway, or vice versa, allowing cells to continue proliferating and surviving. To combat bypass resistance, combination therapies targeting multiple pathways simultaneously are often employed. By inhibiting both the primary target and the bypass pathways, the cells are less able to adapt and maintain their malignant behavior. This approach requires careful selection of drugs and consideration of potential toxicities, but it can be a powerful tool for overcoming resistance.

Furthermore, changes in cellular metabolism can contribute to resistance. Cancer cells often exhibit altered metabolic profiles, allowing them to thrive in conditions of nutrient deprivation or hypoxia. Targeted therapies can sometimes disrupt these metabolic pathways, but cancer cells can adapt by further modifying their metabolism to compensate. For instance, some cancer cells may increase their reliance on glycolysis or oxidative phosphorylation to maintain energy production when a targeted therapy interferes with their primary metabolic pathway. Strategies to address this include combining targeted therapies with metabolic inhibitors that disrupt these alternative metabolic routes. For example, metformin, a commonly used drug for type 2 diabetes, has shown promise in combination with certain targeted therapies by inhibiting mitochondrial respiration. These combination approaches aim to starve the cancer cells of energy and overcome their metabolic adaptations.

Changes in the tumor microenvironment (TME) also play a critical role in resistance development. The TME is the complex ecosystem surrounding cancer cells, consisting of stromal cells, immune cells, blood vessels, and extracellular matrix components. The TME can influence drug delivery, immune responses, and cancer cell behavior. For example, increased angiogenesis (formation of new blood vessels) can lead to increased drug delivery, but it can also create a hypoxic environment that promotes resistance. Similarly, the presence of immunosuppressive cells in the TME can dampen the efficacy of immunotherapies and targeted therapies that rely on immune-mediated killing of cancer cells. Targeting the TME is therefore a promising strategy to overcome resistance. This can involve the use of anti-angiogenic agents to normalize blood vessels and improve drug delivery, or immunomodulatory therapies to stimulate the immune system and overcome immunosuppression. Additionally, drugs that disrupt the extracellular matrix can improve drug penetration and access to cancer cells.

Epigenetic modifications, which are changes in gene expression that do not involve alterations in the DNA sequence itself, can also contribute to resistance. These modifications can alter the expression of genes involved in drug metabolism, DNA repair, or cell survival, leading to resistance to targeted therapies. For example, some cancer cells may silence genes that are required for drug uptake or activate genes that promote DNA repair, making them less susceptible to the drug's effects. Epigenetic drugs, such as histone deacetylase (HDAC) inhibitors and DNA methyltransferase (DNMT) inhibitors, can reverse these epigenetic modifications and restore sensitivity to targeted therapies. These drugs work by altering the structure of chromatin, making DNA more accessible to transcription factors and other regulatory proteins. Combining epigenetic drugs with targeted therapies can therefore be a powerful strategy to overcome resistance.

Finally, the emergence of cancer stem cells (CSCs) can contribute to resistance and disease recurrence. CSCs are a subpopulation of cancer cells that have the ability to self-renew and differentiate into other types of cancer cells. They are often resistant to conventional therapies and can survive treatment, leading to relapse. Targeted therapies that specifically target

CSCs are therefore needed to eradicate this resistant population. These therapies may target signaling pathways that are essential for CSC survival and self-renewal, such as the Wnt, Notch, or Hedgehog pathways. Alternatively, they may target cell surface markers that are specifically expressed on CSCs, allowing for targeted delivery of cytotoxic agents.

In conclusion, overcoming resistance to targeted therapies requires a multifaceted approach that considers the various mechanisms by which cancer cells can evade the effects of these drugs. Strategies include developing next-generation inhibitors that overcome target mutations, combining therapies to block bypass pathways, targeting metabolic adaptations, modulating the tumor microenvironment, reversing epigenetic modifications, and eradicating cancer stem cells. By understanding these mechanisms and implementing appropriate strategies, it is possible to improve the durability of remission and achieve better outcomes for patients.

5 Chapter 5: Lifestyle Factors and Disease Course

The intricate dance between our daily habits and the trajectory of illness is undeniable; what we consume, how we move, and the way we handle stress can significantly influence whether remission becomes a reality. Diet, in particular, acts as a cornerstone, directly affecting inflammation, immune function, and even the gut microbiome—a teeming ecosystem with profound implications for overall health. Understanding and leveraging these lifestyle factors empowers individuals to become active participants in their own health journeys.

Consider the profound influence of diet. We're not simply talking about calorie counting; it's about the quality and composition of our meals. A diet rich in processed foods, saturated fats, and added sugars can fuel chronic inflammation, a known driver of many diseases and a formidable barrier to remission. Conversely, a diet abundant in fruits, vegetables, whole grains, and lean proteins provides the essential nutrients and antioxidants needed to support immune function and cellular repair. Specifically, the Mediterranean diet, characterized by its emphasis on olive oil, fish, nuts, and plant-based foods, has demonstrated remarkable anti-inflammatory effects and is associated with reduced risk of various chronic diseases. But adopting a new dietary pattern isn't just about adding healthy foods; it's also about thoughtfully reducing or eliminating those that contribute to inflammation and disease progression. For some, this might mean limiting red meat and processed meats, while for others, it could involve identifying and eliminating food sensitivities. Remember, dietary changes should be individualized, taking into account specific health conditions, genetic predispositions, and personal preferences.

Exercise isn't just about maintaining a healthy weight; it's a potent modulator of the immune system. Regular physical activity has been shown to enhance immune cell function, improve circulation, and reduce chronic inflammation. Think of exercise as a carefully calibrated medication, with different types and intensities offering distinct benefits. Aerobic exercise, such as brisk walking, running, or swimming, improves cardiovascular health and enhances the activity of natural killer cells, which play a crucial role in destroying virus-infected and cancerous cells. Resistance training, such as lifting weights or using resistance bands, builds muscle mass, which helps regulate metabolism and improve insulin sensitivity. For individuals with chronic illnesses, it's essential to start slowly and gradually increase the intensity and duration of exercise. Consulting with a healthcare professional or a qualified exercise physiologist can help tailor an exercise program to individual needs and limitations. The goal is to find a sustainable exercise routine that you enjoy and that fits into your lifestyle, transforming exercise from a chore into a cherished part of your daily routine.

The subtle yet pervasive impact of stress cannot be overstated. Chronic stress triggers the release of cortisol and other stress hormones, which can suppress immune function, increase inflammation, and disrupt hormonal balance. In essence, stress can undermine the body's natural ability to heal and achieve remission. Learning effective stress management techniques is therefore crucial for supporting overall well-being and enhancing the chances of lasting remission. Mindfulness meditation, for instance, involves focusing your attention on the present moment without judgment, helping to reduce stress, improve focus, and promote a sense of calm. Deep breathing exercises can also be incredibly effective in calming the nervous system and reducing anxiety. Yoga, with its combination of physical postures, breathing techniques, and meditation, offers a holistic approach to stress management. Even simple activities like spending time in nature, listening to music, or engaging in a hobby can provide a welcome respite from the demands of daily life. Identify the stress management techniques that resonate with you and make them a regular part of your routine.

Beyond diet, exercise, and stress management, several other lifestyle factors can influence disease course. Sleep, often overlooked, is essential for immune function, hormonal regulation, and cellular repair. Aim for 7-9 hours of quality sleep each night. Sufficient sleep allows the body to repair and rejuvenate itself, strengthening the immune system and promoting overall well-being. Also, exposure to environmental toxins can impair immune function and contribute to disease progression. Minimize your exposure to pollutants, pesticides, and other harmful chemicals by choosing organic foods, using natural cleaning products, and ensuring good ventilation in your home. Social connection also plays a vital role in health and well-being. Strong social support can buffer against stress, improve mood, and enhance immune function. Spend time with loved ones, join a support group, or volunteer in your community to foster meaningful connections.

Ultimately, the journey towards remission is not a passive one; it requires active participation and a willingness to make meaningful lifestyle changes. While medical treatments play a crucial role, lifestyle factors act as powerful complements, supporting the body's natural ability to heal and achieve lasting remission. By prioritizing a healthy diet, engaging in regular exercise, managing stress effectively, and optimizing other lifestyle factors, individuals can empower themselves to take control of their health and improve their chances of a brighter, healthier future. The interplay of these components provides a harmonized, complete, and effective strategy for disease remission.

5.1 The Impact of Diet on Remission

Our bodies are remarkable machines, constantly working to maintain equilibrium. But what happens when that balance is disrupted by illness? Often, conventional treatments are essential, but they're not the whole story. What we put into our bodies can profoundly influence our ability to achieve and maintain remission. Nutrition isn't just about calories; it's about providing the essential building blocks for cellular repair, immune function, and overall resilience. The connection between food and disease is often underestimated, but it's a powerful tool in our quest for lasting wellness.

Consider the inflammatory response. Many chronic diseases, such as rheumatoid arthritis, inflammatory bowel disease, and even some cancers, are characterized by chronic inflammation. A diet rich in processed foods, sugary drinks, and unhealthy fats can exacerbate this inflammation, hindering the body's ability to heal and potentially preventing remission. Conversely, an anti-inflammatory diet, abundant in fruits, vegetables, whole grains, and healthy fats like omega-3 fatty acids, can help quell this inflammation, creating a more favorable environment for remission to occur. Think of it as tending a garden: you need to nourish the soil (your body) to allow healthy plants (healthy cells) to thrive.

One critical aspect often overlooked is the gut microbiome. Trillions of bacteria, fungi, and other microorganisms reside in our intestines, collectively known as the gut microbiome. This complex ecosystem plays a vital role in digestion, nutrient absorption, immune regulation, and even mental health. An unhealthy diet, high in processed foods and low in fiber, can disrupt the balance of the gut microbiome, leading to dysbiosis. This imbalance can contribute to inflammation, impaired immune function, and increased susceptibility to disease. Probiotics, found in fermented foods like yogurt, kefir, and sauerkraut, can help restore the balance of the gut microbiome. Prebiotics, found in fiber-rich foods like onions, garlic, and asparagus, act as food for beneficial bacteria, promoting their growth and activity. Nurturing our gut is like cultivating a thriving inner garden, one that strengthens our defenses and promotes overall well-being.

Micronutrients are the unsung heroes of remission. Vitamins and minerals, though needed in small quantities, are essential for countless biochemical processes in the body. Vitamin D, for example, plays a crucial role in immune function and bone health, while vitamin C acts as a powerful antioxidant, protecting cells from damage. Deficiencies in these micronutrients can compromise the immune system and hinder the body's ability to heal. A varied and colorful diet, rich in fruits, vegetables, and whole foods, is the best way to ensure adequate intake of micronutrients. In some cases, supplementation may be necessary, but it's important to consult with a healthcare professional to determine the appropriate dosage and avoid potential interactions with medications.

Beyond specific nutrients, mindful eating practices can significantly impact our relationship with food and our ability to manage disease. Eating slowly and deliberately, paying attention to our body's hunger and fullness cues, can help prevent overeating and promote healthy digestion. Mindful eating is also about savoring the flavors and textures of our food, fostering a deeper appreciation for the nourishing power of meals. By cultivating a more conscious relationship with food, we can break free from unhealthy habits and create a sustainable approach to healthy eating.

Navigating the dietary landscape can be challenging, especially with the constant barrage of conflicting information. Fad diets often promise quick fixes, but they are rarely sustainable or healthy in the long run. Instead of focusing on restrictive diets, it's more beneficial to adopt a balanced and personalized eating plan that aligns with our individual needs and preferences. This might involve working with a registered dietitian or nutritionist who can provide evidence-based guidance and support. Remember, there's no one-size-fits-all approach to nutrition; what works for one person may not work for another.

Maintaining a healthy diet during remission isn't just about avoiding certain foods; it's about embracing a lifestyle that prioritizes nourishment and well-being. Cooking at home more often allows us to control the ingredients and preparation methods, reducing our exposure to processed foods and unhealthy additives. Experimenting with new recipes and exploring different cuisines can make healthy eating more enjoyable and sustainable. Furthermore, involving family and friends in meal planning and preparation can create a supportive environment and strengthen our commitment to healthy habits.

The journey towards remission is a marathon, not a sprint. There will be ups and downs, challenges and triumphs. It's important to be patient with ourselves, celebrate small victories, and learn from setbacks. A healthy diet is a powerful tool in our arsenal, but it's just one piece of the puzzle. Other lifestyle factors, such as regular exercise, stress management, and adequate sleep, also play a crucial role in promoting overall health and well-being. By embracing a holistic approach, we can empower ourselves to take control of our health and pave the way for a brighter, healthier future. Remember, food is not just fuel; it's medicine.

5.2 Exercise and Immune Function

Our bodies are intricate machines, and physical activity serves as a master tuner, impacting everything from cardiovascular health to mental well-being. However, the relationship between exercise and the immune system is particularly fascinating, a delicate balance that can either fortify our defenses or, if mishandled, leave us vulnerable. Understanding this interplay is crucial, especially for individuals striving for disease remission, as a well-calibrated exercise regimen can be a powerful adjunct to medical treatments.

For years, the common assumption was that intense exercise invariably suppresses the immune system. Marathon runners, for instance, were often cited as examples of individuals experiencing temporary immune deficits after prolonged exertion, exhibiting increased susceptibility to upper respiratory tract infections. This phenomenon, often referred to as the "open window" hypothesis, suggested that a period of immune compromise followed strenuous activity, creating an opportunity for pathogens to invade. While some evidence supports this concept, painting a picture where exhaustive exercise leads to transient reductions in certain immune cell populations (like natural killer cells and lymphocytes) and altered cytokine profiles, we now understand that this is an oversimplification. The reality is far more nuanced and depends heavily on the intensity, duration, and type of exercise, as well as individual factors like fitness level, age, and overall health.

Let's shift our focus to the positive effects of regular, moderate-intensity exercise on the immune system. Consistent physical activity, such as brisk walking, cycling, or swimming for 30-60 minutes most days of the week, has been shown to enhance immune function in several ways. Firstly, it improves immune cell circulation. Exercise mobilizes immune cells, causing them to circulate more rapidly throughout the body. This enhanced circulation allows immune cells to patrol for pathogens and detect threats more efficiently. Think of it as a neighborhood watch program, where increased patrols lead to quicker detection and response to suspicious activity. Secondly, exercise can stimulate the production of certain immune cells. Regular physical activity may lead to a temporary increase in the number of circulating immune cells, including neutrophils and macrophages, which are crucial for engulfing and destroying bacteria and viruses. Thirdly, exercise has anti-inflammatory effects. Chronic inflammation is a major driver of many diseases, including cardiovascular disease, diabetes, and autoimmune disorders. Regular exercise can help to reduce chronic inflammation by promoting the release of anti-inflammatory cytokines and improving the body's sensitivity to insulin. This reduction in inflammation not only protects against chronic diseases but also allows the immune system to function more effectively.

Navigating the exercise landscape requires careful consideration, particularly for those seeking disease remission. High-intensity workouts, especially if performed infrequently or without adequate recovery, can indeed suppress the immune system, negating the potential benefits. Overtraining, characterized by persistent fatigue, muscle soreness, and decreased performance, is a clear indicator that the body is under excessive stress and the immune system is likely compromised. Conversely, inactivity can also be detrimental, leading to a weakened immune system and increased susceptibility to infections. The key lies in finding the "sweet spot" of moderate-intensity exercise that stimulates the immune system without overwhelming it. Listening to your body is paramount. Pay attention to signs of fatigue, muscle soreness, and illness, and adjust your exercise routine accordingly. When in doubt, err on the side of caution and prioritize rest and recovery. Furthermore, consulting with a healthcare professional or a qualified exercise physiologist is highly recommended, especially for individuals with pre-existing health conditions. They can help you develop a personalized exercise plan that is safe and effective for your specific needs.

Several practical strategies can further optimize the benefits of exercise for immune function. Nutrition plays a crucial role. Ensuring an adequate intake of vitamins, minerals, and antioxidants is essential for supporting immune cell function. A diet rich in fruits, vegetables, whole grains, and lean protein provides the necessary building blocks for a robust immune system. Adequate sleep is equally important. During sleep, the body repairs and regenerates itself, including immune cells. Aim for 7-9 hours of quality sleep each night to allow your immune system to function optimally. Stress management techniques, such as meditation, yoga, or deep breathing exercises, can also help to modulate the immune response. Chronic stress can suppress the immune system, making it more difficult to achieve disease remission. Minimizing stress and cultivating a positive mindset can significantly enhance immune function. Finally, proper hygiene practices, such as frequent handwashing, can help to prevent the spread of infections and reduce the burden on the immune system.

Moreover, it's vital to recognize that exercise is just one piece of the puzzle. While physical activity can significantly boost immune function, it is not a substitute for medical treatments or other lifestyle interventions. It should be viewed as a complementary therapy that works in conjunction with conventional medical care to promote disease remission. Consider the timing of exercise in relation to medical treatments. For example, individuals undergoing chemotherapy may need to adjust their exercise routine to accommodate treatment-related side effects. Working closely with your healthcare team to coordinate exercise with medical interventions is essential for maximizing the benefits and minimizing the risks.

In the quest for disease remission, exercise should be approached as a strategic tool, not a blunt instrument. By understanding the complex interplay between physical activity and the immune system, and by adopting a personalized and holistic approach, individuals can harness the power of exercise to fortify their defenses, improve their overall health, and increase their chances of achieving lasting remission. Think of it as cultivating a vibrant garden, where regular exercise acts as the sunshine and water, nourishing the immune system and allowing it to flourish. It's about finding the right balance, listening to your body, and working in harmony with your healthcare team to create a path towards lasting well-being. Remember, the goal is not to push your body to its limits, but rather to cultivate a sustainable and enjoyable exercise routine that supports your immune system and contributes to your overall health and vitality.

5.3 Stress Management Techniques

The weight of chronic illness extends beyond the physical; it casts a long shadow over mental and emotional well-being, and effective stress management becomes not just a coping mechanism but a vital component of the journey toward remission. Stress, in its various forms, triggers a cascade of hormonal and neurological responses that can negatively impact immune function, cellular repair, and overall physiological balance, thereby hindering the body's natural ability to heal and regenerate. Therefore, integrating strategies to mitigate stress isn't merely about feeling better; it's about creating an internal environment that actively supports the processes of remission. We have to understand that our bodies and minds are in constant communication, a dialogue profoundly influenced by the stresses we endure.

One of the simplest, yet most profound, tools for managing stress is mindful breathing. It's not about emptying your mind, which is often an impossible task, but about gently guiding your attention to the present moment, focusing specifically on the sensation of breath entering and leaving your body. Deep breathing exercises, such as diaphragmatic breathing, can activate the parasympathetic nervous system, often referred to as the "rest and digest" system, which counteracts the effects of the stress response. To practice diaphragmatic breathing, find a quiet and comfortable space where you can sit or lie down without distractions. Place one hand on your chest and the other on your abdomen. As you inhale slowly through your nose, focus on expanding your abdomen, allowing your diaphragm to contract and pull air deeply into your lungs. You should feel your hand on your abdomen rise while the hand on your chest remains relatively still. Exhale slowly through your mouth, allowing your abdomen to gently fall. Repeat this process for 5-10 minutes, focusing on the rhythm of your breath and the sensations in your body. Incorporating this practice into your daily routine, even for just a few minutes at a time, can significantly reduce feelings of anxiety, improve focus, and promote a sense of calm. It's an accessible technique, readily available whenever and wherever stress arises, offering a powerful anchor in the storm of chronic illness. Consistent practice is key to reaping its full benefits.

Another powerful stress-reduction technique involves cultivating a practice of mindfulness and meditation, but it's a more than just sitting cross-legged and chanting. At its core, mindfulness is about paying attention to the present moment without judgment. This can be cultivated through various meditation practices, such as sitting meditation, walking meditation, or even mindful eating. Sitting meditation typically involves finding a comfortable posture, closing your eyes, and focusing on your breath, a sound, or a mantra. When your mind wanders, as it inevitably will, gently guide your attention back to your chosen focus. Walking meditation involves paying attention to the sensations of your feet making contact with the ground as you walk, noticing the rhythm of your body and the surrounding environment. Mindful eating involves savoring each bite of food, paying attention to the textures, flavors, and aromas, and noticing how your body feels as you eat. In my own experience, I've found that even just five minutes of daily meditation can make a noticeable difference in my ability to manage stress and maintain a sense of inner peace. The key is consistency and finding a practice that resonates with you. There are numerous apps and online resources available to guide you through different meditation techniques, making it easier than ever to incorporate mindfulness into your daily life. Remember, it's not about achieving a perfect state of stillness, but rather about cultivating awareness and acceptance of your thoughts and feelings as they arise.

Beyond the internal practices, engaging in regular physical activity, tailored to your individual abilities and limitations, offers profound benefits for stress reduction and overall well-being. Exercise releases endorphins, which have mood-boosting and pain-relieving effects. It also helps to reduce levels of cortisol, the body's primary stress hormone. However, it's crucial to choose activities that you enjoy and that are appropriate for your current health condition. For some, this may mean gentle yoga, tai chi, or swimming, which are low-impact activities that can improve flexibility, balance, and cardiovascular health. For others, it may mean taking a brisk walk in nature, gardening, or simply dancing to your favorite music. I've personally found that spending time outdoors, surrounded by nature, is particularly effective at reducing stress and promoting a sense of calm. The key is to listen to your body and avoid pushing yourself too hard, especially when you're feeling fatigued or unwell. Aim for at least 30 minutes of moderate-intensity exercise most days of the week, but even short bursts of activity can make a difference. Remember, the goal is not to achieve a certain level of fitness, but rather to move your body in a way that feels good and helps to alleviate stress.

Moreover, nurturing strong social connections and engaging in meaningful activities can serve as powerful buffers against stress and isolation. Chronic illness can often lead to feelings of loneliness and disconnection, which can exacerbate stress and negatively impact mental health. Therefore, it's essential to prioritize relationships with loved ones, join support groups, or volunteer your time to causes that you care about. Spending time with people who understand and support you can provide a sense of belonging, reduce feelings of isolation, and offer a valuable source of emotional support. Engaging in activities that bring you joy and purpose can also help to shift your focus away from your illness and toward something positive and meaningful. This may involve pursuing a hobby, learning a new skill, or simply spending time doing things that you enjoy, such as reading, listening to music, or spending time in nature. I've found that connecting with others who are going through similar experiences can be incredibly helpful in managing stress and maintaining a sense of hope. Sharing your struggles and triumphs with others who understand can provide validation, encouragement, and practical advice.

6 Chapter 6: Novel Therapeutic Approaches

The landscape of medical innovation is constantly evolving, pushing the boundaries of what's possible in disease treatment and ultimately, remission. Traditional therapies often fall short in achieving lasting remission, particularly in complex and aggressive diseases. Therefore, exploring novel therapeutic avenues becomes not just desirable, but essential. These new approaches often target the root causes of disease at a molecular level, offering hope for more effective and durable outcomes. We need to be in the constant lookout for options that will help patients to get the remission they are seeking.

Gene editing technologies represent a paradigm shift in therapeutic intervention. At the forefront of this revolution is CRISPR-Cas9, a system derived from bacterial defense mechanisms. This technology allows scientists to precisely target and modify specific DNA sequences within a cell. Think of it like using molecular scissors to cut out a faulty gene and potentially replace it with a corrected version. While applications are diverse and constantly being researched, CRISPR-Cas9 holds immense promise for treating genetic diseases. For example, in inherited disorders like sickle cell anemia or cystic fibrosis, where a single gene mutation is responsible for the disease, CRISPR-Cas9 could potentially correct the defective gene in patient's cells, leading to a functional cure. The technology's potential extends beyond monogenic diseases. Researchers are exploring its use in cancer immunotherapy, where CRISPR-Cas9 could be used to enhance the ability of immune cells to recognize and attack cancer cells. Clinical trials are already underway, evaluating the safety and efficacy of CRISPR-Cas9 in various diseases, and the preliminary results are encouraging. While challenges remain, such as off-target effects (where the editing tool inadvertently modifies DNA sequences other than the intended target) and efficient delivery of the CRISPR-Cas9 system into cells, ongoing research is focused on refining the technology and addressing these limitations. To ensure CRISPR is as efficient as possible, there is the constant need to keep it updated and tested, making sure that the process of using it will be harmless and effective.

Nanotechnology offers a unique approach to targeted drug delivery, addressing a major challenge in traditional chemotherapy and other systemic treatments: off-target toxicity. Conventional drugs often circulate throughout the body, affecting both diseased and healthy cells, leading to significant side effects. Nanoparticles, tiny particles ranging in size from 1 to 100 nanometers, can be engineered to selectively deliver therapeutic agents directly to diseased cells. These nanoparticles can be designed with specific surface modifications that allow them to recognize and bind to unique markers on the surface of cancer cells, for instance. Once bound, the nanoparticles are internalized into the cells, releasing their therapeutic payload. This targeted delivery minimizes exposure of healthy tissues to the drug, reducing side effects and potentially increasing the efficacy of treatment. Researchers are exploring various types of nanoparticles for drug delivery, including liposomes, polymeric nanoparticles, and inorganic nanoparticles. Each type has its own advantages and disadvantages in terms of drug loading capacity, stability, and biocompatibility. Nanotechnology is also being investigated for its potential in diagnostics. Nanoparticles can be used as contrast agents in imaging techniques, allowing for earlier and more accurate detection of disease. For instance, nanoparticles can be designed to accumulate in tumors, making them more visible on MRI or PET scans. The impact of nanotechnology will increase as time goes by, and that will bring an incredible impact to the therapeutic field.

Regenerative medicine seeks to repair or replace damaged tissues and organs, rather than simply treating the symptoms of disease. This field encompasses a range of approaches, including stem cell therapy, tissue engineering, and gene therapy. Stem cells, with their unique ability to differentiate into various cell types, hold tremendous potential for regenerative medicine. Adult stem cells, found in tissues like bone marrow and fat, can be harvested and used to repair damaged tissues in the same individual. Induced pluripotent stem cells (iPSCs), generated by reprogramming adult cells back to a stem cell-like state, offer another source of stem cells for regenerative medicine. iPSCs can be differentiated into any cell type in the body, providing a potentially unlimited source of cells for tissue repair. Tissue engineering involves combining cells, scaffolds (artificial structures that provide support for cell growth), and growth factors to create functional tissues in the laboratory. These engineered tissues can then be implanted into the body to replace damaged or diseased tissues. For instance, researchers have successfully engineered skin grafts, cartilage, and even blood vessels. Gene therapy, as discussed earlier, can also play a role in regenerative medicine by delivering genes that promote tissue repair or regeneration. Regenerative medicine is still a relatively young field, but it holds immense promise for treating a wide range of diseases and injuries, including heart disease, spinal cord injury, and diabetes. Clinical trials are underway to evaluate the safety and efficacy of various regenerative medicine approaches, and the initial results are encouraging. We can see how the future is coming with this type of medicine, and how it will change the way we approach health.

The development and implementation of these novel therapeutic approaches are not without challenges. Gene editing technologies face concerns about off-target effects and ethical considerations. Nanotechnology must address issues of biocompatibility and long-term safety. Regenerative medicine needs to overcome challenges in controlling stem cell differentiation and ensuring proper tissue integration. Furthermore, the cost of these advanced therapies can be prohibitive, raising concerns about accessibility and equity. Overcoming these challenges requires ongoing research, collaboration between scientists, clinicians, and regulatory agencies, and a commitment to responsible innovation. It will require that all parties work together, and that regulations are created to help not only the patients, but also the institutions that want to invest in this kind of field.
Despite these challenges, the potential benefits of these novel therapeutic approaches are undeniable. They offer the promise of more effective and durable remissions, reduced side effects, and improved quality of life for patients. As these technologies continue to advance, they are poised to revolutionize the treatment of a wide range of diseases and transform the landscape of healthcare. The journey towards disease remission is a continuous process of discovery and innovation, and these novel therapeutic approaches represent a significant step forward in this journey. We will constantly be looking for better options, and for ways to improve the lives of the people.

6.1 Gene Editing Technologies

Imagine a world where we could rewrite the very code of life to eradicate disease at its root. Gene editing technologies bring that prospect closer to reality, offering unprecedented precision in manipulating our DNA. However, these tools are not without their complexities, requiring careful consideration and ethical oversight as we explore their potential to pave new avenues for disease remission.

These are not science fiction fantasies anymore; they represent tangible tools being refined and deployed within research settings and, increasingly, clinical trials. Gene editing technologies enable scientists to precisely alter the DNA sequence within cells, essentially correcting genetic mutations that drive disease. Clustered Regularly Interspaced Short Palindromic Repeats, associated with Cas9 (CRISPR-Cas9) is the most well-known of these tools. The CRISPR-Cas9 system functions like a precise pair of molecular scissors, guiding to a specific DNA sequence within the genome, where it makes a cut. This cut then triggers the cell's natural repair mechanisms, which can be harnessed to either disrupt a disease-causing gene or insert a corrected version. But CRISPR isn't the only one, Transcription Activator-Like Effector Nucleases (TALENs) and Zinc Finger Nucleases (ZFNs) are also powerful tools with more difficult handling. For those facing genetic disorders, gene editing offers a glimmer of hope that traditional treatments often cannot provide. Consider sickle cell anemia, a debilitating blood disorder caused by a single mutation in the gene encoding hemoglobin. Gene editing can be used to correct this mutation in a patient's bone marrow stem cells, which then give rise to healthy red blood cells, potentially eradicating the disease. Initial clinical trials have shown remarkable success, with patients experiencing significant reductions in pain crises and improved quality of life. Similar approaches are being explored for other inherited diseases, such as cystic fibrosis and Huntington's disease. However, the long-term effects of these gene editing interventions remain under investigation.

The application of gene editing extends beyond inherited diseases; it also holds tremendous promise for treating acquired conditions, particularly cancer. One strategy involves engineering immune cells, such as T cells, to recognize and attack cancer cells more effectively. This approach, known as CAR T-cell therapy, has already revolutionized the treatment of certain blood cancers. Gene editing can further enhance CAR T-cell therapy by improving the targeting specificity of T cells, making them more resistant to the tumor microenvironment, or preventing them from attacking healthy tissues. Solid tumors present a greater challenge, but researchers are actively exploring novel gene editing strategies to overcome these obstacles.

However, the journey of gene editing from bench to bedside is fraught with challenges. Ensuring the accuracy and specificity of gene editing tools is paramount. Off-target effects, where the editing occurs at unintended sites in the genome, can lead to unforeseen consequences, including the activation of oncogenes or the disruption of essential cellular functions. Researchers are continuously working to improve the precision of gene editing systems and develop robust methods for detecting and mitigating off-target effects. Another challenge lies in delivering gene editing components effectively to the target cells or tissues. Viral vectors, such as adeno-associated viruses (AAVs), are commonly used for gene delivery, but they can elicit immune responses and have limited cargo capacity. Non-viral delivery methods, such as nanoparticles and electroporation, are also being explored as alternatives.

Ethical considerations are at the forefront of the gene editing debate. Germline editing, which involves making changes to DNA that are passed on to future generations, raises particularly complex ethical concerns. While germline editing could potentially prevent inherited diseases from being passed down, it also carries the risk of unintended consequences and raises questions about the modification of the human gene pool. Most countries have strict regulations or bans on germline editing for reproductive purposes. Somatic cell editing, which involves making changes only to the cells of a particular individual, is generally considered to be more ethically acceptable, as the changes are not heritable. However, even somatic cell editing raises questions about informed consent, access to treatment, and the potential for unintended consequences.

Looking ahead, the future of gene editing holds immense potential for transforming medicine and paving new avenues for disease remission. As the technology continues to advance, we can expect to see more precise, efficient, and safe gene editing tools emerge. Personalized gene editing strategies, tailored to the unique genetic makeup of each patient, will become increasingly common. The integration of gene editing with other innovative therapies, such as immunotherapy and regenerative medicine, holds promise for tackling complex diseases that are currently incurable.

Furthermore, the development of new delivery methods will expand the reach of gene editing to a wider range of tissues and organs. Researchers are exploring the use of exosomes, naturally occurring vesicles secreted by cells, to deliver gene editing components to specific locations in the body. Microfluidic devices, which can precisely control the flow of fluids at the microscale, are also being developed to facilitate gene editing in a high-throughput and controlled manner.

As we navigate this exciting new frontier, it is crucial to engage in open and transparent discussions about the ethical, social, and regulatory implications of gene editing. Clear guidelines and regulations are needed to ensure that gene editing technologies are used responsibly and ethically, and that the benefits are shared equitably across society. Education and public engagement are also essential to foster informed decision-making and address public concerns about gene editing.

Gene editing stands as a testament to human ingenuity and our unwavering pursuit of better health. While challenges remain, the progress made in recent years has been nothing short of remarkable. As we continue to refine these technologies and grapple with the ethical considerations they raise, we can look forward to a future where gene editing plays a central role in preventing and treating a wide range of diseases, ultimately leading to lasting remission and improved quality of life for countless individuals.

Gene editing is not a magic bullet, but a powerful tool that, when wielded responsibly, has the potential to reshape the landscape of medicine and leave a lasting legacy of lustre for generations to come.

6.2 Nanotechnology for Targeted Drug Delivery

Imagine a microscopic army, not of soldiers, but of nanoparticles, each carrying a potent payload designed to seek out and destroy disease at its source. This is the promise of nanotechnology in targeted drug delivery, and it's a rapidly evolving field with the potential to revolutionize how we treat a wide range of illnesses, offering the tantalizing possibility of durable remission. For beginners, understanding this field can seem daunting, but breaking it down into fundamental concepts makes it accessible and inspiring.

At its core, targeted drug delivery aims to improve the therapeutic index of a drug – that is, to maximize its effectiveness while minimizing its side effects. Traditional drug delivery methods often result in systemic exposure, meaning the drug circulates throughout the body, affecting both healthy and diseased tissues. This can lead to significant side effects and limit the dosage that can be safely administered. Nanotechnology offers a solution by creating delivery systems that can selectively target diseased cells or tissues, concentrating the drug where it's needed most and sparing healthy areas. Think of it as a guided missile versus a shotgun blast. The guided missile hits its target with precision, minimizing collateral damage.

The building blocks of this technology are nanoparticles, typically ranging in size from 1 to 100 nanometers. These tiny structures can be made from a variety of materials, including lipids (fats), polymers (long chains of molecules), metals, and even biological materials like proteins or DNA. The choice of material depends on the specific application, considering factors like biocompatibility (how well the body tolerates the material), biodegradability (how easily the material breaks down), and the type of drug being delivered. For example, liposomes, spherical vesicles made of lipid bilayers, are often used to encapsulate water-soluble drugs, protecting them from degradation and allowing them to circulate longer in the bloodstream. Polymeric nanoparticles, on the other hand, can be engineered to release their drug payload slowly over time, providing sustained therapeutic effects. Metallic nanoparticles, such as gold nanoparticles, can be used for imaging and diagnostics, as well as for delivering drugs and therapeutic genes.

The magic of targeted delivery lies in the ability to engineer these nanoparticles with specific targeting ligands – molecules that bind to receptors or other markers that are overexpressed on the surface of diseased cells. These ligands act like address labels, guiding the nanoparticles to their intended destination. For instance, in cancer therapy, nanoparticles can be decorated with antibodies that recognize proteins found only on cancer cells. This allows the nanoparticles to selectively bind to and enter cancer cells, delivering their cytotoxic payload directly to the tumor. Another common targeting strategy involves exploiting the enhanced permeability and retention (EPR) effect. Tumor blood vessels are often leaky, allowing nanoparticles to passively accumulate in the tumor microenvironment. Furthermore, tumors often lack effective lymphatic drainage, which further contributes to nanoparticle retention. By designing nanoparticles within the appropriate size range (typically 20-200 nm), they can preferentially accumulate in tumors via the EPR effect.

Once the nanoparticles reach their target, they need to release their drug payload. This can be achieved through a variety of mechanisms, including changes in pH, temperature, or enzyme activity. For example, some nanoparticles are designed to release their drug cargo in the acidic environment of a tumor cell's lysosomes. Others can be triggered to release their payload by external stimuli, such as light or ultrasound. This allows for precise control over drug release, further enhancing the therapeutic effect and minimizing side effects. Consider a scenario where chemotherapy drugs are encapsulated in nanoparticles that are sensitive to the lower pH found within cancer cells. As these nanoparticles are internalized by the tumor, the acidic environment triggers the release of the chemotherapy drug, selectively killing cancer cells while sparing healthy tissues.

The applications of nanotechnology in targeted drug delivery are vast and expanding. In cancer therapy, nanoparticles are being used to deliver chemotherapeutic drugs, gene therapies, and even radiation therapy directly to tumors. In infectious diseases, nanoparticles can deliver antibiotics or antiviral drugs to infected cells, improving their efficacy and reducing the risk of resistance. In inflammatory diseases, nanoparticles can deliver anti-inflammatory drugs directly to the site of inflammation, minimizing systemic side effects. Gene therapy is another promising area where nanotechnology can play a crucial role. Nanoparticles can be used to deliver therapeutic genes to cells, correcting genetic defects and potentially curing inherited diseases.

However, challenges remain in translating these promising technologies from the lab to the clinic. One major challenge is the biocompatibility and toxicity of nanoparticles. While many nanoparticles have been shown to be safe in preclinical studies, their long-term effects on human health are still not fully understood. Another challenge is the scale-up of nanoparticle production. Many nanoparticle formulations are complex and difficult to manufacture on a large scale, which can limit their availability and increase their cost. Finally, there are regulatory hurdles to overcome. Nanoparticles are a relatively new class of therapeutic agents, and regulatory agencies are still developing guidelines for their approval.

Despite these challenges, the field of nanotechnology for targeted drug delivery holds immense promise for the future of medicine. As researchers continue to develop new and improved nanoparticles, and as regulatory agencies become more familiar with these technologies, we can expect to see a growing number of nanoparticle-based therapies entering the clinic.

The ultimate goal is to develop therapies that are more effective, less toxic, and more personalized, offering the hope of durable remission for a wide range of diseases. I believe that through continued research and development, we can unlock the full potential of nanotechnology to transform healthcare and improve the lives of millions. It's a journey worth embarking on, a testament to human ingenuity in the face of disease.

6.3 The Promise of Regenerative Medicine

Regenerative medicine stands as a beacon of hope, offering the tantalizing prospect of not merely treating diseases but actually reversing their effects and restoring tissues and organs to a state of youthful functionality. It's a field built upon the body's innate capacity for healing, amplified and directed with sophisticated techniques to address conditions that were once considered irreversible. For the newcomer, grasping the core concepts is key to appreciating its transformative potential. We are talking about the possibility of healing by means of cells and cell-based technologies, and this brings a world of possibilities.

Central to regenerative medicine is the concept of harnessing the power of cells. Stem cells, with their remarkable ability to differentiate into various cell types, are a cornerstone of this approach. Think of them as blank slates, capable of becoming specialized cells like heart muscle, nerve tissue, or insulin-producing pancreatic cells. Sourcing these cells can be done in a number of ways. Embryonic stem cells, derived from early-stage embryos, possess the highest regenerative potential, but their use raises ethical concerns that necessitate careful consideration. Adult stem cells, found in various tissues throughout the body, offer a more readily accessible and ethically less contentious alternative. These cells, however, often have a more limited differentiation capacity compared to their embryonic counterparts. A third major source is induced pluripotent stem cells (iPSCs), which are adult cells that have been reprogrammed to behave like embryonic stem cells. This groundbreaking technology sidesteps the ethical dilemmas of embryonic stem cells while offering a high degree of pluripotency.

Beyond stem cells, regenerative medicine also encompasses other cell-based therapies. This involves using mature, specialized cells to repair or replace damaged tissue. For instance, cartilage cells can be harvested from a patient's own knee, grown in a lab, and then implanted back into the knee to repair cartilage damage. Similarly, skin grafts, using a patient's own skin cells, are a standard treatment for severe burns, effectively regenerating damaged skin. But even with the advancements that are being done every day, scientists have to consider some factors. Scaffolds and biomaterials provide structural support and guidance for cells to grow and regenerate tissues. These scaffolds can be made from a variety of materials, both natural and synthetic, and can be designed to degrade over time as the new tissue grows, leaving behind a fully functional, regenerated organ or tissue. Growth factors, signaling molecules that stimulate cell growth and differentiation, are also critical components of regenerative medicine strategies. By delivering growth factors to the site of injury or disease, scientists can encourage cells to proliferate and rebuild damaged tissues.

Applying these principles in practice is where the true excitement lies. For example, in the field of cardiology, researchers are exploring the use of stem cells to regenerate damaged heart tissue after a heart attack. The goal is to replace the dead or scarred tissue with healthy, functional heart muscle, thereby improving heart function and preventing heart failure. In diabetes, regenerative medicine offers the potential to replace or regenerate insulin-producing pancreatic cells, potentially eliminating the need for insulin injections. Researchers are investigating various approaches, including transplanting engineered pancreatic cells or stimulating the regeneration of existing pancreatic cells. Neurodegenerative diseases, such as Parkinson's and Alzheimer's, are also targets for regenerative medicine strategies. The hope is to replace or repair damaged nerve cells in the brain, thereby slowing or even reversing the progression of these debilitating diseases. Spinal cord injuries, which can lead to paralysis, are another area of intense research. Scientists are exploring ways to regenerate damaged spinal cord tissue and reconnect severed nerve pathways, potentially restoring movement and sensation.

Despite the incredible promise, it's important to acknowledge the challenges and limitations that regenerative medicine still faces. One major hurdle is the complexity of tissue engineering. Recreating the intricate structure and function of complex organs like the liver or kidney is an enormous challenge, requiring precise control over cell differentiation, organization, and vascularization. Immune rejection is another significant concern. When cells or tissues from a donor are transplanted into a recipient, the recipient's immune system may recognize them as foreign and attack them, leading to graft rejection. Overcoming this requires careful matching of donor and recipient tissues and the use of immunosuppressant drugs, which can have side effects. The regulatory landscape for regenerative medicine is still evolving. Because these therapies often involve living cells, they pose unique challenges for regulatory agencies like the Food and Drug Administration (FDA). Clinical trials must be carefully designed to ensure the safety and efficacy of these novel therapies, and the long-term effects must be closely monitored.

Yet, the field continues to advance at an astonishing pace. New technologies are constantly emerging, pushing the boundaries of what's possible. Bioprinting, for example, allows scientists to create three-dimensional structures using cells and biomaterials, potentially paving the way for the creation of artificial organs. Gene editing technologies, such as CRISPR-Cas9, offer the possibility of correcting genetic defects that contribute to disease, opening up new avenues for regenerative therapies. As research continues and technologies mature, regenerative medicine is poised to revolutionize healthcare, offering hope for cures and improved quality of life for patients suffering from a wide range of diseases.

7 Chapter 7: The Future of Disease Remission

The horizon of disease remission is not a static line but a dynamic, ever-evolving landscape sculpted by relentless innovation and a deepening understanding of the human body. We stand at the cusp of a transformative era where diseases, once considered intractable, are increasingly yielding to the power of scientific advancement. Central to this future is the convergence of data, technology, and biological insight, promising a paradigm shift in how we diagnose, treat, and ultimately, achieve lasting remission. Artificial intelligence is poised to revolutionize diagnostics in ways we can scarcely imagine today. Instead of relying solely on subjective interpretations of medical images or traditional lab tests, expect AI-powered algorithms to sift through vast datasets of patient information, identifying subtle patterns and anomalies that would escape the human eye. Imagine a scenario where a routine blood test, analyzed by an AI, detects the earliest signs of recurrence, months or even years before conventional methods. This capability extends beyond oncology, impacting the diagnosis of autoimmune disorders, infectious diseases, and even neurological conditions. This isn't just about faster results; it's about uncovering hidden connections and individual risk profiles with unparalleled precision, enabling proactive interventions tailored to each patient's unique circumstances. Moreover, the ability of AI to continuously learn and adapt from new data ensures that diagnostic tools remain at the cutting edge, constantly refining their accuracy and expanding their capabilities. Early detection can be a game-changer in the fight against disease progression, offering hope for remission.

The potential of predictive modeling extends far beyond early diagnosis. Think of it as a crystal ball, not to predict the future deterministically, but to estimate the likelihood of different outcomes based on a complex interplay of factors. By feeding AI algorithms with comprehensive patient data – genomic information, lifestyle factors, environmental exposures, treatment responses – it becomes possible to create personalized risk assessments and predict how a patient might respond to different treatment options. For instance, imagine a newly diagnosed cancer patient receiving a predictive model that assesses the probability of remission with different chemotherapy regimens, taking into account their individual genetic makeup and tumor characteristics. This allows clinicians to make more informed decisions, avoiding ineffective treatments and minimizing unnecessary side effects. Furthermore, predictive modeling can optimize clinical trial design, identifying patient subgroups who are most likely to benefit from a particular therapy and accelerating the development of innovative treatments. This data-driven approach is about transitioning from a one-size-fits-all approach to a highly personalized strategy, where treatment is tailored to the individual's unique disease biology and predicted response. It is about understanding the complex system of interactions that contribute to disease progression and relapse, and using that knowledge to proactively steer patients toward remission.

As we venture deeper into the realm of personalized medicine and advanced technologies, ethical considerations become paramount. The vast troves of patient data required for AI-driven diagnostics and predictive modeling raise concerns about privacy, security, and potential misuse. We must ensure that data is collected, stored, and used responsibly, with robust safeguards to protect patient confidentiality and prevent unauthorized access. The potential for bias in AI algorithms is another critical ethical challenge. If the data used to train an AI model is skewed or reflects existing health disparities, the resulting predictions could perpetuate and even exacerbate those inequalities. To mitigate this risk, we need diverse and representative datasets, along with careful monitoring and validation of AI algorithms to ensure fairness and equity. Moreover, as technology advances, we must address the issue of accessibility. The benefits of AI-driven diagnostics and personalized medicine should not be limited to wealthy individuals or privileged communities. We must strive to make these innovations accessible to all, regardless of socioeconomic status, geographic location, or other factors. This requires concerted efforts to reduce costs, develop user-friendly technologies, and train healthcare professionals in underserved areas. The ethical use of these technologies is not just a matter of compliance but a moral imperative to ensure that technological advancements benefit all of humanity.

Consider also the psychological and emotional impact on patients. Knowing one's predicted risk of relapse, even if it is only a probabilistic assessment, can create anxiety and uncertainty. It is crucial to provide patients with adequate counseling and support to help them navigate this information and make informed decisions about their care. Open and transparent communication is essential, explaining the limitations of predictive models and emphasizing that they are not deterministic prophecies. The ultimate goal is to empower patients to take an active role in their health management, not to instill fear or create a sense of helplessness. The future of disease remission is not just about technological advancements, it is about fostering a collaborative and compassionate partnership between patients and healthcare providers, leveraging technology to enhance human connection and improve the overall quality of care.

As personalized medicine continues to evolve, patients should expect to see an increasing number of targeted therapies that exploit unique vulnerabilities in their disease. These therapies might include gene editing tools that directly correct the underlying genetic defects driving disease or nanotechnology platforms that deliver drugs with unparalleled precision to diseased cells. Regenerative medicine approaches may also play a role in restoring damaged tissues and organs, ultimately achieving lasting remission. This multi-pronged approach, combining advanced diagnostics, personalized therapies, and regenerative strategies, represents a truly revolutionary shift in how we approach disease management.

We must remember, achieving lasting disease remission is not solely about technological breakthroughs. It is also about fostering a holistic approach to health that encompasses lifestyle factors, preventive measures, and patient empowerment. Diet, exercise, stress management, and other lifestyle interventions can play a crucial role in modulating the immune system, reducing inflammation, and promoting overall well-being, thereby increasing the likelihood of remission. By educating and empowering patients to take control of their health, we can create a more resilient and proactive healthcare system that prioritizes prevention and early intervention. The convergence of technology, personalized medicine, and holistic health practices will pave the way for a future where disease remission is not just a possibility but a tangible reality for millions of people around the world. This future hinges on our collective commitment to innovation, ethical responsibility, and a relentless pursuit of knowledge, ensuring that the benefits of scientific progress are shared equitably across all of humanity. It is a future where the legacy of lustre shines brightly, illuminating the path toward a healthier and more hopeful world.

7.1 Artificial Intelligence in Diagnosis

The integration of computational power into the diagnostic process represents a paradigm shift, particularly in the pursuit of lasting remission.

We're not just talking about faster lab results; instead, we're envisioning a comprehensive, AI-driven system that analyzes vast amounts of patient data – from genomic sequences to lifestyle habits – to provide personalized diagnoses and predict individual responses to treatment. This proactive approach moves beyond simply identifying a disease to predicting its trajectory and tailoring interventions for optimal remission.

Think of a patient newly diagnosed with leukemia. Traditionally, diagnosis relies on a bone marrow biopsy, microscopic examination, and standard cytogenetic testing. However, even with these tools, subtle variations in the disease that might impact treatment response can be missed. Here's where AI steps in. By applying machine learning algorithms to large datasets of leukemia patients, including their genetic profiles, treatment regimens, and outcomes, an AI system can identify patterns and predict how this specific patient will respond to different therapies. It can flag potential resistance mutations early on, suggesting alternative treatment strategies from the outset. I believe this type of informed decision-making dramatically increases the likelihood of achieving deep and durable remission, minimizing relapse and improving the patient's overall quality of life.

The power of AI extends beyond predicting treatment response. Consider the challenge of diagnosing rare diseases, many of which manifest with subtle and non-specific symptoms. A child experiencing unexplained developmental delays, for example, might undergo a lengthy and frustrating diagnostic odyssey involving multiple specialists and a battery of tests. AI-powered diagnostic tools can accelerate this process. By inputting the child's symptoms, family history, and initial test results into an AI system trained on a vast database of rare disease information, clinicians can generate a prioritized list of potential diagnoses. The system can highlight specific genetic mutations or metabolic markers that warrant further investigation, leading to earlier and more accurate diagnoses. In such cases, time is of the main essence. Early diagnosis can unlock opportunities for targeted therapies or supportive care that can significantly improve the child's prognosis and quality of life. Imagine the relief and hope this could provide to families desperate for answers.

However, the true potential of AI in diagnosis lies in its ability to integrate and analyze diverse data streams. We now have access to an unprecedented amount of information about each patient – from electronic health records containing medical history, lab results, and imaging studies, to wearable sensors tracking activity levels, sleep patterns, and even vital signs. AI can act as a central nervous system, integrating and making sense of this information. Consider a patient with rheumatoid arthritis. AI can analyze their blood test results for inflammatory markers, their imaging studies for joint damage, and their activity data from a wearable sensor to assess their level of disability. This holistic view allows clinicians to tailor treatment plans more effectively, optimizing medication dosages, physical therapy regimens, and lifestyle interventions to achieve and maintain remission.

The development of these AI diagnostic tools requires careful consideration of several key factors. First, the quality and quantity of data are paramount. AI algorithms are only as good as the data they are trained on. Therefore, it is essential to create large, well-curated datasets that accurately reflect the diversity of the patient population. Secondly, it is essential to address the issue of bias in data. If the data used to train an AI system is biased towards certain demographic groups, the system may perform poorly for patients from other groups. Addressing this bias requires careful attention to data collection and preprocessing, as well as the development of algorithms that are robust to bias. A final, important consideration is the ethical implications of AI-driven diagnosis. We need to ensure that these tools are used responsibly and that patients are not discriminated against based on AI-generated predictions. This requires clear guidelines for the use of AI in healthcare and a commitment to transparency and accountability.

My personal experience in the field has shown me the human element remains vital. AI is a tool, not a replacement, for clinical judgment. The best approach is a collaborative one, where AI provides insights and recommendations, but the ultimate decision-making remains in the hands of the healthcare professional. It's about augmenting human expertise, not supplanting it. This collaborative model ensures that the patient's individual needs and preferences are always at the forefront of care.

In conclusion, AI holds immense promise for revolutionizing disease diagnosis and improving the chances of achieving lasting remission. By analyzing vast amounts of patient data, predicting treatment responses, and accelerating the diagnosis of rare diseases, AI can empower clinicians to make more informed decisions and tailor treatments for optimal outcomes. As we move forward, it is essential to address the challenges related to data quality, bias, and ethical considerations to ensure that AI-driven diagnosis is used responsibly and equitably for the benefit of all patients. Ultimately, AI will be a transformative force in the future of medicine, offering hope for achieving enduring remission and enhancing the quality of life for individuals living with chronic diseases.

7.2 Predictive Modeling for Patient Outcomes

Predictive modeling represents a pivotal shift in our approach to disease management, moving beyond reactive treatment strategies to proactive, personalized interventions. It's about leveraging the power of data to anticipate patient trajectories, predict treatment responses, and ultimately, enhance the likelihood of achieving and maintaining disease remission. I believe that this field will reshape how we deliver healthcare.

The foundation of predictive modeling lies in the availability and integration of diverse data sources. Consider the vast amounts of information generated in modern healthcare systems: electronic health records (EHRs) containing patient demographics, medical history, lab results, imaging reports, and medication lists; genomic data providing insights into individual predispositions and disease mechanisms; lifestyle data gathered through wearable devices and patient surveys; and even environmental data reflecting exposure to pollutants or other risk factors. The challenge, and the opportunity, lies in harmonizing these disparate datasets into a cohesive, analyzable form. Data warehousing techniques and standardized data formats are crucial for this process. Without clean, well-organized data, even the most sophisticated algorithms will produce unreliable predictions. This isn't just about collecting information; it's about curating a comprehensive picture of each patient.

Once the data is prepared, the selection of appropriate modeling techniques becomes paramount. Several options exist, each with its own strengths and weaknesses. Statistical regression models, such as logistic regression and Cox proportional hazards models, are relatively simple to implement and interpret. They can identify statistically significant associations between predictor variables and outcomes, such as the probability of achieving remission or the time to relapse. However, they may struggle to capture complex, non-linear relationships. Machine learning algorithms, including support vector machines, random forests, and neural networks, offer greater flexibility in modeling complex interactions. These algorithms can learn from large datasets without explicit programming, potentially uncovering subtle patterns that would be missed by traditional statistical methods. Yet, the complexity of machine learning models can also make them difficult to interpret, raising concerns about transparency and trust. The best approach often involves a combination of techniques, using simpler models to identify key predictors and more complex models to refine the predictions. A critical step is also cross-validation to avoid overfitting the model to a limited dataset. Overfitting results in excellent performance on the training data but poor generalization to new patients. Model evaluation is an ongoing process. Key metrics include accuracy, sensitivity, specificity, and area under the receiver operating characteristic curve (AUC-ROC). Accuracy measures the overall correctness of the predictions, while sensitivity indicates the ability to correctly identify patients who will achieve remission (true positives), and specificity indicates the ability to correctly identify patients who will not (true negatives). The AUC-ROC provides a comprehensive measure of the model's ability to discriminate between these two groups. However, it's important to recognize that no model is perfect. There will always be some level of error, and the goal is to minimize the consequences of these errors. For example, in the context of disease remission, a false negative prediction (predicting that a patient will not achieve remission when they actually will) might lead to a missed opportunity for aggressive treatment, while a false positive prediction might lead to unnecessary interventions. The relative costs and benefits of different types of errors should be carefully considered when evaluating model performance.

The integration of predictive models into clinical workflows presents a significant challenge. It's not enough to simply develop a model; it must be seamlessly integrated into the decision-making process. This requires the development of user-friendly interfaces that present predictions in a clear and actionable manner. For instance, a physician might see a patient's predicted probability of remission displayed prominently in their EHR, along with a list of factors that are driving that prediction. The system could also generate personalized treatment recommendations based on the model's output. However, it's crucial to avoid "black box" models that provide predictions without any explanation. Physicians need to understand the reasoning behind the predictions in order to trust them and incorporate them into their clinical judgment. Explainable AI (XAI) techniques can help to address this issue by providing insights into the model's decision-making process. Moreover, education and training are essential to ensure that healthcare professionals understand how to use predictive models effectively and responsibly. It's also important to remember that predictive models are just one tool in the clinician's toolbox. They should not replace clinical judgment but rather augment it, providing valuable insights that can inform decision-making.

Beyond individual patient predictions, predictive modeling can also be used to identify broader trends and patterns in disease remission. By analyzing data from large populations, researchers can identify factors that are consistently associated with successful outcomes. This can lead to the development of new interventions and prevention strategies. For example, a predictive model might reveal that patients who adhere to a specific diet and exercise regimen are more likely to achieve lasting remission. This information could then be used to develop targeted lifestyle interventions for at-risk patients. Predictive modeling can also be used to optimize the allocation of healthcare resources. By identifying patients who are at high risk of relapse, healthcare providers can prioritize them for more intensive monitoring and support. This can help to prevent costly hospitalizations and improve overall outcomes. Furthermore, analyzing treatment patterns and patient responses can help healthcare systems to identify the most effective and cost-effective strategies for achieving remission.

I think it is essential to consider the ethical implications of predictive modeling. The use of sensitive patient data raises concerns about privacy and security. It's crucial to implement robust data governance policies and security measures to protect patient information from unauthorized access. Moreover, predictive models can perpetuate existing biases if they are trained on data that reflects historical inequalities. For example, a model that predicts remission rates based on socioeconomic status might inadvertently reinforce disparities in healthcare access and outcomes. It's important to carefully evaluate the data used to train predictive models and to ensure that they are fair and unbiased. This may involve techniques such as data augmentation, which involves adding synthetic data to the training set to address imbalances. It also requires ongoing monitoring of model performance to identify and correct any biases that may emerge over time. Transparency and accountability are essential to building trust in predictive models.

In conclusion, predictive modeling holds tremendous promise for improving patient outcomes in the context of disease remission. By leveraging the power of data and sophisticated algorithms, we can move towards a more proactive, personalized, and effective approach to disease management. However, realizing this promise requires careful attention to data quality, model selection, clinical integration, ethical considerations, and continuous evaluation. I am excited to see how this field evolves and the positive impact it will have on the lives of patients.

7.3 Ethical Considerations and Accessibility

The pursuit of lasting disease remission brings with it a constellation of ethical responsibilities and the crucial imperative of ensuring equitable access to advancements. We're venturing into a landscape where the potential to alter disease trajectories is becoming increasingly tangible, and with it comes the duty to navigate the complex moral terrain these possibilities create. How do we ensure that the transformative power of medical progress benefits all, regardless of socioeconomic status, geographic location, or any other arbitrary barrier? This is the central question we must address.

The rising dependence on intricate technologies for diagnosis, personalized treatment plans, and continuous monitoring introduces several ethical dilemmas. Sophisticated algorithms and predictive models, for instance, can offer valuable insights, but they also run the risk of perpetuating existing biases present in the data they are trained on. Consider, for example, a predictive model designed to identify individuals at high risk of relapse. If the data used to train this model disproportionately represents a certain demographic group, the model may inaccurately flag individuals from other groups, leading to unequal treatment and reinforcement of health disparities. Similarly, the use of gene editing technologies raises profound questions about the limits of medical intervention and the potential for unintended consequences. While these technologies hold promise for correcting genetic defects that drive disease, we must proceed with caution, ensuring that these powerful tools are used responsibly and ethically. Robust oversight mechanisms and transparent data practices are paramount to mitigating these risks and maintaining public trust.

Accessibility to innovative treatments stands as a major challenge. Advanced therapies, such as gene editing and personalized immunotherapy, often carry exorbitant price tags, making them unattainable for many patients, particularly those in underserved communities. This economic barrier exacerbates existing health inequalities and creates a two-tiered system where access to life-altering treatments depends on financial capacity. A comprehensive strategy to address this challenge requires a multipronged approach. Government subsidies, public-private partnerships, and innovative pricing models are essential to lower the cost of these therapies and ensure that they are available to all who need them. Furthermore, we must invest in infrastructure and training in underserved areas to ensure that these communities have the capacity to deliver advanced treatments effectively. Telemedicine and mobile health technologies can also play a crucial role in expanding access to care, particularly for patients in remote or rural locations.

The importance of informed consent in the context of novel therapies cannot be overstated. As we push the boundaries of medical innovation, it is essential that patients fully understand the potential risks and benefits of participating in clinical trials or receiving cutting-edge treatments. Informed consent should not be a mere formality but a dynamic process that empowers patients to make autonomous decisions about their own healthcare. This requires clear and concise communication, culturally sensitive educational materials, and access to independent counseling services. Furthermore, researchers and clinicians must be vigilant in protecting patient privacy and confidentiality, particularly when dealing with sensitive genetic information.

Looking ahead, the integration of patient-reported outcomes (PROs) into clinical research and healthcare delivery holds immense promise for improving the quality of care and ensuring that treatments are aligned with patient needs and preferences. PROs provide valuable insights into the patient's lived experience with a disease, including their symptoms, functional status, and overall well-being. By incorporating PROs into clinical trials, we can gain a more comprehensive understanding of the impact of different treatments on patients' lives. Moreover, PROs can be used to monitor patients' progress over time and identify those who may be at risk of relapse or disease progression. This information can then be used to tailor treatment plans and provide timely interventions to improve patient outcomes.

The concept of "remission equity" must become a guiding principle in our pursuit of disease control. This means actively working to eliminate disparities in remission rates across different populations. This requires a commitment to addressing the social determinants of health, such as poverty, lack of access to education, and environmental factors that can contribute to disease risk. It also requires culturally tailored interventions that are designed to meet the specific needs of diverse communities. For instance, outreach programs that provide education about disease prevention and early detection can be particularly effective in reaching underserved populations. Similarly, community-based clinics that offer affordable and accessible healthcare services can help to reduce health disparities.

Finally, the ethical dimensions of utilizing stored biological samples and patient data for research purposes necessitate careful consideration. These resources, often collected during routine clinical care or past research endeavors, represent a treasure trove of information that can accelerate our understanding of disease mechanisms and identify new targets for therapy. However, their use raises important questions about patient privacy, data security, and the potential for commercial exploitation. Clear guidelines and regulations are needed to ensure that these resources are used responsibly and ethically, with appropriate safeguards in place to protect patient interests. This includes obtaining informed consent from patients for the use of their samples and data, ensuring that data is anonymized or de-identified to protect patient privacy, and establishing transparent governance structures to oversee the use of these resources. We stand at the cusp of a new era in disease management, one where remission is not just a possibility, but an attainable goal for many. Let us proceed with wisdom, compassion, and a steadfast commitment to ethical principles and equitable access. The legacy we leave should be one of lasting lustre, not just in scientific achievement, but in the unwavering pursuit of justice and well-being for all. The journey towards disease remission should be inclusive, ensuring that no one is left behind.

www.ingramcontent.com/pod-product-compliance
Lightning Source LLC
LaVergne TN
LVHW022011200926
848481LV00007B/2327